Journey to a Healthier Me

A travel guide for physical & emotional
well-being after weight loss surgery

by Pam Tremble

Ordering Information:
Quantity sales. Special discounts are available on quantity purchases by corporations, associations, and others. Book signings and appearances can be arranged directly with the author. For details, contact Pam Tremble at the address above or by calling (989) 284-3110.

www.PamTremble.com/Journey

Printed in the United States of America

Pam Tremble. Journey to a Healthier Me: A travel guide for physical & emotional well-being after weight loss surgery

ISBN: 978-0-9888310-0-1

Dedication

To my family for your unwavering support of everything I do or try. You don't care how much I weigh, how farfetched my goals may seem, how silly I might act, or how grumpy I might get, you support me no matter what and I can't thank you enough. I love you all!

To my WLS support groups, friends, blog readers, and the rest of the amazing bariatric community for always being there when I need someone to lean on. You have made this journey more enjoyable than you know.

To Dr. Jamal Farhan, Dr. Gerard Williams, Linda Krueger, the entire staff at Hurley Bariatric Clinic and the rest of my medical team. Thank you for your outstanding work, support, patience, and expertise.

To Nikki for your enthusiastic cheerleading, contributions to my sanity with your chatter, educating me about passive voice, and your willingness to kick my butt when I need it.

To Mikey for believing in me.

Contents

Abbreviations

RNY	Surgery type: Roux-en-Y Gastric Bypass
Band	Surgery type: Adjustable Gastric Band
Sleeve	Surgery type: Vertical Sleeve Gastrectomy
DS	Surgery type: Biliopancreatic Diversion with Duodenal Switch
WLS	Weight Loss Surgery (the medical term is bariatric surgery)
Pre-op	A weight loss surgery patient, before surgery
Post-op	A weight loss surgery patient, after surgery
Non-op	Everyone else in the world who didn't have weight loss surgery

Introduction
The story of Pam's journey

On November 13, 2007 I had Roux-en-Y gastric bypass surgery. This is the story of my journey to health. Just like most of us, over-eating and under-exercising is what brought me to morbid obesity. But when I was ready to lose the excess weight, I discovered I was facing an insurmountable task that I couldn't tackle on my own. With a diagnosis of Polycystic Ovarian Syndrome (PCOS), which came along with insulin resistance and a hormonal imbalance, my body simply would not allow me to lose the weight I tried so hard to shed.

After years of failed dieting, exercise that made little difference, and the advice of my ill-informed family doctor to "just try harder," I was at the end of my rope. I knew I needed medical intervention.

Both my sister and my mother had Roux-en-Y several years before me, so I knew the success I could have with the surgical option. But I also knew the drastic changes and sacrifices I would need to make in my life and it took me a long time to come to the realization that I was willing and able to make those changes.

I spent several months seriously contemplating the decision and researching my options. I made lists upon lists – lists of pros and cons of having surgery in the first place; then lists of pros and cons for each type of surgery available; lists of the diets I'd tried and which things worked or didn't work; lists of questions I had; lists of what things I wanted to research; lists of doubts and fears that were holding me back; task lists and thinking lists and lists of goals and great things I could accomplish after surgery. (I'm a bit of a list person.)

Once all the tasks were checked off my lists, I was left with the actual decision to make. I needed to find some quiet time to think.

The morning of August 5, 2006 I got in my car and drove. I ended up at a roadside park just outside Port Austin, Michigan – about 90 minutes from my house. I made my way down to the narrow strip of beach and sat on an old piece of driftwood that had washed up onto shore years ago. After two hours of solitude, soul searching, and a few shed tears, I made the final decision to go ahead with surgery.

I consulted with a bariatric surgeon and realized that with medical intervention I finally had a real option to get healthy and with his help, decided that Roux-en-Y gastric bypass surgery was the right option for my circumstances. The next step was to get insurance approval. That approval process took nearly a year and a half, which gave me plenty of time to be 110% sure it was the right option for me.

It was a quick recovery from surgery, and then the real work began. Imagine suddenly having the stomach of a newborn infant and needing to learn how to drink, chew, and swallow food as if you were a baby. Calling it a lesson in humility and experimentation is an understatement. Within six weeks after surgery I was off all medications for high blood pressure, asthma, and allergies. I was finally able to sleep through the night, my chronic back pain vanished and the symptoms of my PCOS were slowing going away too.

To me this journey has always been about more than just losing weight. Being skinny was never the goal. Being healthy and having the opportunity to live a longer, happier life has been my main focus. I have set many other "life goals" that have nothing to do with the number on a scale or how many miles I can walk or what size jeans I can fit into.

Shortly after my surgery I enrolled in a ten-week group therapy class for bariatric patients. One exercise in the sessions gave us the opportunity to create our own Comprehensive Holistic Wellness Plan. I set goals that focused not only on my physical health, but also my emotional, spiritual, financial, intellectual and vocational health, the health of my relationships, and my overall character.

Having a written plan for all areas of my life has helped me stay focused on what is really important and what I want to achieve – not only as it relates to my weight loss surgery (WLS) journey, but also for how I want to live my life and how I want to transform the person I am now into what I want to be while pursuing my ultimate purpose in life. I recommend you use WLS as the springboard for making all the changes you want to see in your life, not just your physical health.

Three months after my surgery I hesitantly signed up for a 20-week walking training program which included a 10-mile road race and a 13.1-mile half marathon at the end of the training. I signed up with a huge doubt hanging over my head. "How can a morbidly obese person ever hope to finish a half marathon?" But even with the doubts, I just put one foot in front of the other and transformed myself into Walker Girl.

I was walking an average of 60-80 miles every month and slowly the hesitation about my ability to walk a half marathon grew into a confidence that the finish line was squarely within my realm of reality. And yes, I crossed both finish lines before I hit my one-year surgery anniversary.

A huge unanticipated benefit of weight loss surgery is the friendships I have developed along the way. I attend three different support group meetings each month where members of the WLS community gather to help each other through the struggles and celebrate the triumphs of the journey. After attending the peer-based support group in my hometown for a year and a half, the members asked me to be their new leader, I graciously accepted. Now I'm able to help new surgery patients find their way and encourage the old timers to stay on track. The bonds of friendship are strong in the community and I'm a better person for having these people in my life.

I started my blog on the day I officially decided to have WLS. I believe that by keeping a written journal of my experiences I have been more accountable to myself and it's given me a written record of my day-to-day life over time, giving me a clearer picture of where I started and how far I've come.

When I started my blog I made the commitment to be honest and forthright about what was going on with my life. I didn't want to show just the fun and exciting part of the bariatric experience. I wanted my journal to be a true picture of my experiences — the good days and the bad days, the struggles and the victories, the detailed nutritional research I would dig up, advice and guidance from those going before me, healthy recipes, my exercise challenges, my life goals and the triumphs I've experienced along the way.

Throughout the years, my blog has become one of the most important tools I've used on my journey. Please visit: **www.PamTremble.com/Journey**

Because my surgery of choice was Roux-en-Y, much of the information contained here is gear toward that type of surgery. However, the basic guidelines for post-op life apply to all four surgery types with only slight variations that may be specific to your surgery. I often say, and passionately believe, that the

WLS journey is about 10% the physical surgery we receive and the other 90% is about getting our heads screwed on straight, establishing a healthy relationship with food, and learning to love yourself enough to do the healthy thing for your body and mind.

Please keep in mind that in this writing, when I say the word "pouch" I'm actually referring to all our pouches universally – the sleeved and/or banded stomachs have many of the same characteristics as the RNY pouch. Obviously, those with an exclusively restrictive surgery (Vertical Sleeve Gastrectomy and Adjustable Gastric Band) can skip over any information about malabsorption of calories or nutrients as that information does not apply to your specific surgery type.

Although many of the lessons in this book apply directly to WLS patients, there is plenty of information for our non-op friends (those who did not have weight loss surgery and are attempting to lose weight through diet and exercise alone). Because I believe that our physical bariatric surgery is only about 10% of the process of losing weight and keeping it off, the other 90% of the process is an emotional journey to becoming a healthier person. So share this book and what you learn with your non-op friends, as well.

Please remember, though, that I am not a medical professional and have not received any formal medical training. I'm not a nurse, doctor, or nutritionist. I'm simple a bariatric patient with a thirst for knowledge, a desire to share what I've learned, and a drive to help others as they navigate the path to better health through bariatric surgery. If you have any medical or technical questions or concerns, I advise you to consult your medical team for assistance.

When I look at all the goals I have achieved so far I know that I am a success and life can only get better and better. RNY has given me the opportunity to change my life and I'm so much happier for the hard work I've put into the journey. I wish you the same happiness.

Chapter 1
Is Surgery Right for You?

So you're thinking about having weight loss surgery. This is a huge decision you're about to make - one that cannot be taken lightly because it will affect every aspect of your health for the rest of your life. It's a journey of a lifetime. A journey to a healthier you.

What many people don't realize is this journey of health doesn't begin on the day you have weight loss surgery (WLS). It begins months before your surgery date is even scheduled. Not only must you decide if surgery is right for you, but you must also determine how you're going to pay for surgery and which surgeon you'll entrust with this life changing operation. And there are a thousand other decisions to be made too.

- What should you do first and how soon should you do it?

- What is a priority and what can wait until later?

- What can you expect to happen along the way?

Even if you're only "kinda-sorta" thinking about bariatric surgery right now, follow these steps while you continue to think about it. Do not wait until you have decided one way or the other – do these steps right now. And do it in this specific order. If you're already out of order on these steps, go back to the beginning and do the steps you have missed so far.

Why do I think it's so important to follow these steps in order? The reason it took 16 months for my surgery to be approved is because I didn't do this part right. If I had followed these steps, I would have been approved in just a couple months. I'm laying out these specific steps for you so you can avoid the agonizing and frustrating delays I experienced.

Because I didn't insist my primary doctor properly document my dieting attempts in my medical chart, I was required to start over and do the diet history a second time. My insurance company required, at the time, a 12-month physician supervised diet – that requirement has since changed. By the time I had my Roux-en-Y (RNY) surgery, I'd done a straight 24 months of physician supervised dieting – twice as long as required by my insurance company – all because the first 12 months were not documented correctly. So please, learn from my mistake.

Step 1 - Start a physician-supervised diet today

First, get an appointment with your primary care physician (PCP). Call today and set this appointment for as soon as you can get in. Once you have set this appointment, move immediately on to Step 2 before you arrive at your doctor's office.

At the appointment with your doctor, explain to him that you want to pursue bariatric surgery. Explain that you're in the research phase, but that you understand your insurance company will likely require some type of documented weight loss attempts supervised by a physician. Show him the information you gathered in Step 2 and be sure he has a copy of these requirements for his files. He'll likely need to order various tests in the coming months as you obtain medical clearance for surgery so be sure he understands what his role will be in this process.

Ask for his support and be sure he's on board with your decision. You'll need a doctor who is supportive of bariatric surgery and willing to treat your special needs after surgery — this initial appointment will be your gage for his level of supportiveness. Even if he's not supportive, still start the diet documentation and you can deal with the doctor situation later (yes, I recommend you find a new primary care physician who is supportive of bariatric surgery if yours is not). Your medical records travel with you if you change doctors, so be sure this visit is properly documented even if you don't have support from your current doctor.

At this initial appointment, you will discuss your dieting attempts of the past and what you will do in the future. Ask for your doctor's recommendation on which food plan you should follow — what nutrient balance and caloric limits your diet should have and discuss what behavioral changes you'll be making including your exercise plan, psychological or nutrition counseling, food logging, etc. It doesn't matter which diet you follow, it matters that you're discussing it and that your doctor is writing it down in your medical chart, including the start date and the dates of any subsequent appointments where you discuss your weight loss attempts. Be sure he documents your weight, your BMI, blood pressure and whatever other information is required by your insurance company guidelines. Get it all in writing.

Some insurance companies require monthly visits. If yours does, then work with his office staff to get all follow up appointments set exactly one month apart so you don't miss any appointments and have to start over.

Step 2 - Call your insurance company

Do this when you get off the phone with the receptionist at your PCP's office and have the answers before you see your doctor. Call the number on the back of your insurance card and before you start asking questions, make sure they ask you for your policy number and identify you by name. This ensures they are telling you information based on your specific policy and what is covered under your plan.

Here are the questions you need to ask:

1. Is bariatric surgery a covered procedure? Do not call it weight loss surgery. Do not call it a treatment for obesity. Call it bariatric surgery because that is the medical term for the procedure and some insurance policies have specific language that prevents "treatment for obesity" - but we know that WLS is not a treatment for obesity, it's a treatment for our co-morbidities, or the medical conditions that result from obesity. If bariatric surgery is covered, proceed with the remaining questions. If surgery is not covered – don't fret, this is not the end of the road. Ask why it is not covered. If there is an exclusion on your policy, request that a copy of that specific language be sent to your home address so you can double-check the information before you pursue other payment or legal options.

2. What types of bariatric surgery are covered? Know all of the different surgeries your insurance covers even if you don't think you'll consider all of them. The four main types of surgery currently being performed include: Roux-en-Y Gastric Bypass; Adjustable Gastric Band; Vertical Sleeve Gastrectomy and Biliopancreatic Diversion with Duodenal Switch.

3. What are the criteria for insurance approval for each of the surgeries? Is the criteria the same for all or are there specific requirements for some that don't apply to others? The criteria that you'll likely hear include (as outlined by the National Institutes of Health):

- Candidates should have a body mass index (BMI) of 40 or higher.

- Candidates with a BMI between 35 and 40 — surgery may be considered if they have co-morbidities such as cardiopulmonary issues, severe sleep apnea, diabetes, metabolic syndrome, etc.

- Physician supervised diet attempts to include regular weigh-ins, diet and behavioral changes, exercise therapy, pharmacological considerations, etc.

- Psychological evaluation

- Medical clearance based on specific co-morbidities

- Medical history (2 to 5 years) indicating chronic morbid obesity

4. Does your insurance require that you use a Bariatric Center of Excellence or a surgeon who is in-network? Or may you choose whomever you want to for your surgery? You may also want to ask about your specific co-pay requirements or any out-of-pocket expenses you might be expected to pay.

After you hear the specific information from the insurance representative on the phone, get a copy of these exact criteria in writing. Some insurance companies have their policy available on their website — if so, ask the representative to walk you through the website to find the section while you're on the phone so you can print a hard copy. If it's not available online, ask for a hard copy to be mailed to your home - this might take a couple weeks, but that's alright, as long as you get a hard copy of these guidelines in the your hands.

This document will become your checklist for fulfilling the criteria and sharing with your primary care physician.

Do not rely on anyone else to get this information for you. Your primary care physician or surgeon's office may also have access to this information through their computer billing system, but be sure you have your own copy obtained directly from your insurance carrier and keep it for your records and reference. Again, this is a mistake that I made and relied on information I obtained from my surgeon's office, which omitted the importance of the documented diet attempts.

Share copies of this information with your PCP and your surgeon to make sure everyone is working from the same checklist throughout the process. Your surgeon may also have additional requirements for surgical approval, so be prepared to discuss those items as well.

These requirements for surgical clearance and insurance approval may seem cumbersome and overwhelming. I know that when you're ready to have bariatric surgery, you're ready "right now"—you don't want to have to jump over a bunch of hurdles to get to your goal. But these requirements are in place for a reason. Bariatric surgery comes with many surgical and post-surgical risks - not only because it is major surgery, but also because any type of surgery performed on morbidly obese patients comes with additional risk factors. There are also considerable psychological pressures put upon WLS patients as they make major life changes after surgery.

These myriad requirements are designed to make sure we are in the absolutely best health possible before we have surgery. Doctors want us to survive and be successful. So think of these requirements as a way for you to have the best chance at success on your journey to better health.

Also remember that each insurance policy is different. That's why it is essential that you get the exact requirements from your own insurance company's representative and not rely on word of mouth from other patients or friends. Even if you have the same insurance company as someone else, your policy may still not be the same as someone else's. Each employer negotiates their own policy with the insurance company. And some employers offer a type of insurance coverage menu so employees can choose the type of policy that works best for their individual and family needs.

Step 3 - Start your research

Notice that this is Step 3 on the list. That's by design. Those first two things need to happen before you decide to have surgery or not. If you're even thinking about it a little bit, get those first two steps done right now!

There are countless resources available that give you a history of obesity and why it is such a terrible disease. Even studies that theorize why we're facing an obesity epidemic in the United States and around the world and what we can do about it. Because this topic is so well covered elsewhere, I won't go into the details of obesity as a general topic here.

There are also countless resources available that will guide you through the process for choosing the right bariatric surgery for you. Because of these resources, I will not cover those details within the scope of this writing.

However, as you are researching bariatric surgery, keep these several things in mind. First, remember that there are four main types of bariatric surgery being performed today. Here is a list:

Roux-en-Y Gastric Bypass (abbreviated as RNY)
Restriction and malabsorption

Adjustable Gastric Band (abbreviated as band or the brand name LapBand)
Restriction only

Vertical Sleeve Gastrectomy (abbreviated as Sleeve)
Restriction only

Biliopancreatic Diversion with Duodenal Switch (abbreviated as DS)
Restriction and malabsorption

Learn about all four surgery types even if you don't think you're interested in them. Do the research and keep an open mind. Know as much as you can about each one and understand which one is the right fit for you — they are all good surgeries, but not all are good for every person. Each surgery type has a "personality" of its own and you need to find the surgery that fits you as a person both physically and emotionally.

Take the time to do an in-depth self-examination and try to match yourself with the best surgery for you. Think about the following as you do this self-exam:

- Which diets have I tried in the past?

- Why did those diets fail?

- What are my trigger foods and how will surgery change that?

- What is the cause of my obesity? (hint: the answer to this question is not "because I like to eat.")

- Why do I overeat? How will my surgery choice change that?

- Am I unable to lose weight no matter which diet I attempt? If so, had my doctor identified the reason why?

- Do I struggle with controlling portion sizes or is the struggle more related to the foods I choose to eat? Or both?

- Am I able to lose weight on my own but struggle to keep it off for the long term?

- Do I have an underlying food addiction or obsessive compulsive disorder that has contributed to my morbid obesity? (hint: almost all of us have one or the other to some degree and a therapist can help)

There are also medical considerations to think about when looking at the different types of bariatric surgery. What medical issues do you have that can be resolved with surgery? What is the expected resolution of those medical conditions for each of the surgery types? (i.e.: Type 2 Diabetes is resolved in 95% of DS patients, 80% of RNY patients, and only 56% of gastric band patients.[1])

As you begin your research, there are two books I highly recommend you read cover-to-cover (preferably more than once). These two books together will help guide you through your decision making process — which surgery to choose based on your own personal habits, medical considerations and goals as well as how to choose a surgeon and bariatric clinic. They will also help prepare you for what life is like post-op in terms of eating, follow-up care and how to handle the emotional challenges that come along with the whole journey. I wish both of these books would be required reading for every WLS patient before they were allowed to have surgery (and yes, I've told my own surgeon this too).

Weight Loss Surgery for Dummies
by Marina S. Kurian, Barbara Thompson, Brian K. Davidson

The Emotional First Aid Kit: A Practical Guide to Life After Bariatric Surgery
by Cynthia L. Alexander

Read, read, read and then read some more! Read as much as you can get your hands on. Not just books and magazines about WLS, but also the stories of those who are living the life. I started my blog on the day I decided to have bariatric surgery in 2006 and I chronicled my journey through the insurance maze, life leading up to surgery, and through the many adventures after my surgery. There are others who have done the same thing. Find those people, read their stories, and learn from their experiences (see Resources section).

So I'll say it again. Read, read, read... and when you think your eyes are going to fall out, read some more. That's my mantra. Really. I've read more since I started my weight loss surgery journey than I've ever read in my life. But the more I read, the more I learn.

And don't just read the good stuff. Read the scary stuff, read about complications and death rates, about the emotional battles, and regaining the weight — know what others struggle with and how they overcame those struggles. Find out what life is like in the real world of weight loss surgery, not just what you learn at the informational seminars at your surgeon's office.

Read forums dedicated to bariatric patients who are several years out from surgery; understand what challenges they are facing each day and how they work through those daily battles. Learn from them. Soak it all up. Even if you don't think something applies to you, read it anyway, learn it now and tuck it away in a back corner of your mind... because one day, it might apply to you and by knowing others have experienced it before you, it will help you to be prepared to deal with it if it does happen to you. So go read – learning is fun!

Google is your friend. I'm not going to insult your intelligence by giving you a step-by-step guide to using Internet search engines. We all know how to use Google and many people, like me, are self-professed "Googleheads." Some interesting things you might want to search for include:

- Stories, websites and blogs of other bariatric patients, bariatric surgeons, obesity experts and even nutritional researchers and scientists

- Forums and online chat rooms where the WLS community gathers

- Websites for bariatric clinics around the world who publish their patient post-op guide books, patient newsletters, recipes or tips for their own patients

- Information about nutrition, digestion and how your body's anatomy works with various vitamins, minerals and macronutrients

There's also a really cool feature on Google that many people don't know about. It's called Google Scholar which is a section of Google's main search engine that only searches professional publications like the New England Journal of Medicine or associations like the American Society of Bariatric and Metabolic Surgeons (and thousands of other trade publications and associations for countless industries).

You might not be able to get to full reports on some publications without a subscription to that specific trade journal, but there is plenty of information there that you can read. And if you find an abstract summary you want to read more fully, contact your local library for help in obtaining the full version of the study. This handy search engine allows you to see what the scientists are saying about bariatric surgery and what their studies are telling us right now. For this type of research you're going to need your thinking cap and a good dictionary ... but it's worth the effort.

Step 4 - Interview Surgeons and Clinics

First, decide how far you're willing to travel to see your surgeon or how far is too far for an emergency. Some people feel comfortable traveling out of state or out of the country whereas some prefer a doctor who is close to home – you'll need to decide what your comfort level is with distance from your bariatric team. I personally wanted my surgeon close - within a one hour drive. Thankfully within that one hour distance, I had several top surgeons to choose from.

Now that you know your target area, make a list of all the bariatric surgeons in your immediate area. Then start researching the individual surgeons on your list and attending their free informational seminars (nearly all clinics have these). Attend as many as you need to attend until you find the surgeon and clinic that is right for you.

It is important to find a good surgeon with a good record and lots of skill and training – and plenty of experience. But remember that the surgeon is really only important for the first day of your journey when you're on the operating table.

You must also take a very close look at the aftercare you'll receive and the clinic where that surgeon practices. These are the questions you need to be thinking about as you choose a surgeon and clinic. Surgery lasts one day... aftercare is forever.

- Do they have support group meetings? Are the meeting times convenient for your schedule?

- Is there a nutritionist on staff and available for your every question (and there will be a lot of them)?

- Are there a psychologist and medical doctor associated with the clinic that is available to patients? There are psychologists who specialize in the treatment of bariatric patients and have a better understanding of what we face and how to use us. Medical doctors who specialize in caring for WLS patients are called bariatricians.

- Is the nursing staff knowledgeable, friendly and accessible?

- Does the clinic want to see you annually for the rest of your life or do they only care about the first 90 days?

- What is the success rate of the clinic as a whole?

- What is the complication rate?

- Is the office staff attentive, friendly and prompt in returning calls?

Step 5 - Join the Community

I attended a local support group for 15 months before I had my surgery. Because I feel these meetings are essential to my success, I make them a priority in my life and rarely miss a meeting. Find a support group — whether it's peer-based or medical-based — and attend regularly. Add the meetings to your calendar and commit to faithfully attending each and every month.

Make friends, ask questions and listen to their advice. An in-person support group is essential, in my opinion, for successful long term weight maintenance. But don't just take my word for it. Studies have shown that patients who attend support group meetings see a 10% higher rate of weight loss over those who do not attend.[2]

Also join an online community. There are dozens of different online forums to choose from. I've visited many of the different online forums, but I was most comfortable at ObesityHelp.com. It is an excellent resource and support, but there are many others and each online community has their own personality, so find the one that fits you best.

Many online forums have various sub-forums to join — get involved in your local state forum and make friends (this is also a great way to find local in-person support group meetings). There are also forums for the specific surgery type you've chosen or forums for various special interests in other parts of your life (scrapbooking, photography, sports, or dating).

Surround yourself with the people who understand what you're going through and know how to help you through the process. And stay surrounded. This is an exciting and terrifying journey. If you get started in the right direction from the beginning ... it will be less scary and more exciting.

Chapter 2
Preparing for Surgery

You're approved for weight loss surgery and you have your official surgery date. Congratulations! Now you're faced with the agonizing weeks of waiting.

This is usually the time when people start to freak out a bit. All the work to get your insurance approval has given you a specific goal and a narrow focus. But now that you are facing the reality of actually having your surgery and starting this new chapter in your life, the emotions start to set in. Fear, worry, nervousness, excitement, anticipation, impatience — you're going to feel all those things and many, many more. This is all normal. If you weren't scared or nervous, then I'd be concerned for you. Bariatric surgery is a huge step, so I expect you to be scared of the life changes you're about to make.

The key to holding on to your sanity in the last few weeks before surgery is to rest assured that you're doing the right thing… but also to stay busy and keep your mind on all the stuff that needs to get done before the big day. The suggestions that follow should help you be as prepared as possible for life after surgery.

Start a journal

In fact, start two journals. The first journal will be an accounting of this exciting and amazing journey you're embarking upon. The changes are going to come at you fast and furious — faster than you can anticipate. There is no way for you to remember all the amazing things that are about to happen unless you document them in some way.

This can be a paper journal and your favorite pen; markers, paint, and crayons in an art journal; or it can be an online journal that's either public or private (you know I'm partial to the blogging option). Or it can simply be a section in your WLS Bible (see below). It doesn't matter what form your journal takes, but it is an essential part of this exciting new journey.

Without my own place to write I might have missed the opportunity to create my Wow List – which is a list of all the little things I experienced along the way that made me say, "Wow!" And when I say little things, I really do mean little. Like being able to cross my legs for the first time, or fit into a booth at a restaurant and having room to spare, or moving the driver's seat forward a notch because my belly shrank. These little moments need to be recorded, so start your list and keep it going.

No matter what method you use for your journal, start thinking about it now and get a system in place for capturing all the fun stuff about to happen.

The second journal is going to be part of your emotional therapy. An Emotional Journal is a place for you to write your most private thoughts about the emotional hurdles you face on this journey to better health. Here you will explore the reasons you became obese in the first place, dig into your innermost thoughts to repair your relationship with food and with the loved ones in your life and have a safe place to express any thought that's crowding your mind. This WLS journey is an emotional roller coaster and you'll need to deal with the mental stuff that will creep into your everyday life.

Just as with the first journal, you can choose any media that feels comfortable to you. I actually have two different emotional journals, one is a paper journal that I can write in longhand and the other is a file on my computer where I can type my thoughts in a document that's grown to several hundred pages.

Start your WLS Bible

I have a regular old three-ring binder where I keep all the information about my own personal weight loss surgery journey. I have a copy of my medical records, a listing of all my current medications (including dosage, prescribing doctor, reason for taking it, etc.), my personal reasons for wanting WLS and a list of my goals. I also have a copy of all the paperwork my surgeon's office gave me including the checklist of requirements I needed to fulfill before surgery, letters from my insurance and PCP, my physician-supervised diet documentation, etc.

As a handy reference, I keep a copy of the nutrition book I received from my nutritionist that includes my eating plan and sample menus. I keep my weight chart and measurements chart in this binder along with copies of all my lab results.

Each section is concise and well organized. I take this book with me to all doctor appointments and keep it on my kitchen counter for easy access and reference. Even now, many years post-op, this binder goes with me to all my doctor appointments and is regularly updated with new information as I receive it.

Continue your research

Now your research is going to change focus slightly. You've already researched the reasons for having surgery and the overview of what will happen to your body afterward. But now you need to dig deeper and learn the nitty-gritty of the details. A starting point might be:

- How are certain vitamins and supplements going to affect your body? Why are certain supplements better for us than others?

- How are medications processed in your new body? Will you need to change your prescriptions after surgery?

- What are the differences in types of exercise and what is best for your body type, limitations, and physical abilities? How will those exercises change once you begin losing weight and become more physically fit?

Another important aspect of your research will feel like you're reliving high school biology class. Study the human digestive system and understand the path food takes and how the body breaks down food and processes it into fuel and new cell development.

Then once you understand how your anatomy works with an intact digestive tract, learn how that anatomy changes with the surgery type you've chosen. Which parts are cut or altered and how are those parts disconnected or reconnected? What new path does food take and how does it intermingle with digestive enzymes?

I don't mean to scare you with the science part of this surgery. And you don't need to dig so deep into this biology lesson that you feel like you're studying for medical school. But you do need to understand your anatomy enough that if you're ever in the emergency room faced with a doctor who doesn't understand how your altered body works, you can explain it to them and maybe even draw them a sketch of your innards. A basic understanding of your newly altered anatomy is essential.

Start collecting recipes

There are millions of recipes to be found online and in various healthy-cooking cookbooks. But when you narrow your search to recipes that have been created and tested by bariatric patients you'll find a whole new world of recipes that you never knew existed.

One of the big benefits of being part of the WLS community is the sharing of recipes that happens between veteran post-op patients and newbie post-op patients. It's awe inspiring and exciting to learn the healthy ways to prepare some of our favorite comfort foods from the past.

For instance, you'll find healthy ways to eat pizza, cheesecake, mozzarella sticks, ice cream and even lasagna. Yes, really! With a few alterations and ingredient substitutions all these foods are perfectly legal after WLS — and absolutely delicious. You'll also find recipes that are specific to your post-op stage of eating. For instance, in the early weeks after surgery you'll be restricted to full liquids or soft/pureed foods and there are myriad recipes available that fit those restrictions.

As you stumble across these types of recipes, save them! Print a copy and create a notebook or save the website link into a favorites folder or copy/paste the recipe to a word processing document to refer to later.

There are several ways to find these recipes. Within the online communities there are often daily discussions surrounding accountability for food and exercise. One I participated in is called "What are you eating/doing today?" — each morning dozens of people post their day's meal and exercise plans. Along with these meal and snack lists will come recipes or links to recipes that people find along the way. This type of discussion is also helpful in planning your own meals for the day because you'll see what other people are eating who are about the same "post-op-age" as you.

Clean house

This section might seem a bit obvious, but yes, I'm literally advising you to clean your house. Chase away the dust bunnies and spit-polish every square inch. Catch up on the laundry and change the sheets on every bed in the place. Scrub the toilets, wax the floors and clear the clutter.

Why? Because after surgery you are going to be on strict lifting and activity restrictions for several weeks and you'll be recovering from major surgery, which means sitting around doing a whole lot of nothing. By cleaning your house before surgery, you'll be less tempted to overexert yourself and cause injury while you're recovering. Most surgeons won't let you lift more than five pounds for a full six weeks and will restrict your level of movement — twisting, bending, reaching — for that same time frame. So get cleaning!

Now is also the time to clear out the pantry and kitchen cupboards of any foods you won't be eating after surgery (or shouldn't be eating before surgery while trying to lose weight). Give it to family members or a food bank — get it out of the house. The sooner you get rid of temptations the easier it'll be to stick to your pre-op diet plan.

Take a critical look at your dishware

I got rid of my huge pasta bowls and oversized plates and any other dishware that promoted oversized servings. Take a critical look at what is in your cabinets and decide which items can stay and which must go. Not only will downsizing your dinnerware sizes help you eat smaller portions, it'll also help your family focus on healthier portion sizes too. Keep your salad and dessert-sized plates since these will be the perfect size for your post-op meals and snacks. But maybe it's time to push the full size dinner plates to the back of the cabinet or save them for non-WLS guests or family members.

After I got rid of all my oversize dishes, I then started shopping around for new dishes that were smaller and that I'd enjoy using for my meals. You don't need to buy new dishes for your surgery, but personally I felt this was an important task for me.

Once I found the dish set I liked, instead of buying the big dinner plates and bowls for these new dishes, I only bought the salad plates and dessert size bowls. I bought these for myself after I was approved for surgery as a congratulatory gift to myself for dealing with all the insurance hoops. Then I didn't start using them until after I came home from the hospital after surgery. They're pretty and make me happy when I eat off them and it reinforces the fact that I'm completely changing my way of eating - not just the food is different, even the dishes are different.

Consider your disposable dishes, too

Yes, I'm about to get scolded by the environmentalists in the room. I spent nearly ten years of my career life as a professional tree hugger, environmental education manager, and "Garbitch" — so I understand the advice I'm about to give is not politically correct or environmentally friendly. But it'll make the time following your surgery easier and less stressful. We can save the planet another day. For now, we need to focus on making life as easy as possible in the weeks following major life-altering surgery.

Protein shakes are messy and make washing glasses very difficult if you don't rinse them right away. I, personally, drink my protein shakes on the run most often (on my 90-minute commute to work each morning) — and leaving a glass in the car all day and trying to get it clean the next day is a pain in the neck. So I opted for disposable plastic cups for my protein shakes.

I also chose to use disposable plastic storage containers in the early weeks after my surgery — the five ounce size with a lid that you can purchase at a large restaurant supply store (i.e.: Sam's Club, Costco or Gordon Food Service).

Why do I think these are important too? While on the full liquid diet you'll be eating a lot of cream soups or pureed foods, but when you prepare these foods you won't be able to eat it all in one sitting — one can of cream soup will last six meals in the first weeks after surgery and it's easier to store the leftovers in individually portioned containers. Then you can easily grab a pre-portioned container for the next meal. At the end of the week you're going to have a lot of leftovers that you won't be eating.

So unless you have family members who are excited about eating cream of mushroom soup or pureed peas, you'll likely be throwing away some food. But you aren't going to feel like washing dishes as you recover from surgery. So it's easier to just toss the whole bowl in the trash instead of washing twenty tiny Tupperware containers when all you really want to do is take a nap. I had enough to worry about in the early days after surgery; I didn't want housework to be one of them. Stock up on some disposable containers to make life easier.

Clean the closet

You will be shrinking out of clothes faster than you can comprehend once you start losing weight. Take the time before your surgery to assess what clothes you have in your closet and clear out what you no longer need or want. Get rid of any clothes that are in your current size but out of season or something you wouldn't wear in the next two months anyway. Also dig through those stored boxes of "skinny clothes" in the back of the closet and organize what you currently own. Make sure your closet is organized and ready for change — because change is a-comin'.

Start a clothing fund

Once I started losing weight, I was caught off guard by how quickly I dropped clothing sizes. I had several smaller sizes in the back of my closet but I blew through sizes so fast that I found myself with very little to wear within a couple months after surgery. I had to find a way to restock my closet without draining my bank account. Thrift stores, yard sales, begging from friends and borrowing clothes from family members helped get me through the rapid size change and kept clothes on my back. But what about that whole new wardrobe you're going to need once you finally reach your goal weight or settle into a consistent size of clothes?

Start a clothing fund! I heard this suggestion from a surgery-veteran before my surgery and I'm so glad I did it. Here's how it works.

At the end of each pay period I would clean out my wallet of whatever cash I had left (usually just a few ones and maybe a five) and add it to my clothing fund jar. Anytime extra money would come my way, it would be added to the clothing fund jar. This might be a few dollars repaid to me from a loan to a friend or a rebate check from something I purchased or a gift card received for the holiday — it all went into the clothing fund jar.

As I was collecting dollars and quarters over the course of the first year after surgery I never counted how much money was in the jar. I wanted to take the entire lump sum and go on a shopping spree when I hit my goal weight and buy whatever I wanted for myself. And once I made the leap from saving to spending it was so much fun to know that every piece of clothing I bought was a reward for a job well done!

Find a support group

I've mentioned this before, but it bears repeating. An in-person support group is the most important thing I've done for myself. The information shared at a peer-to-peer support group is invaluable. You hear what others are struggling with as well as the suggestions from a dozen other people about how they overcame that same particular struggle. This is real-life stuff here! I've made some great friends, have learned from those who have gone before me and have been able to help others by sharing my own experiences. I learn something every single time I go to a meeting. If you haven't already found a support group, now is the time to get involved.

Buy your vitamins

In the weeks leading up to your surgery your bariatric team will provide you a list of the vitamins they want you to start taking after surgery (some practices have you start taking vitamins before surgery). There are dozens of different brands on the market and the choices can become overwhelming. And to add to the confusion about which brand to choose, there are specific restrictions and requirements you need to consider when choosing the right vitamins for your post-op body. Thankfully there are guidelines for you to follow when making this big decision and we'll go over those guidelines in greater detail later in the book.

Buy a 7-day pill organizer

They aren't just for forgetful senior citizens anymore (sorry Grandma!). Because we take a large variety of vitamins each day — in several doses throughout the day — having a system for organizing your supplements is essential. I have found for myself, and I've heard from countless other post-op patients, that a 7-day pill organizer is the easiest way to stay on track with the vitamins.

I sort my vitamins into these organizers — one for morning vitamins, one for evening. Then each morning I dump my morning vitamins into a smaller daily pill box that I carry with me and take my doses of vitamins at my scheduled times. By using a daily pill organizer, it makes it easy to remember to take my required vitamins and know at a glance which doses I've taken and which still need to be done.

Find some protein supplements

It is common in most bariatric programs for patients to use some type of protein supplement after surgery. Some surgeons recommend using a supplement for only the first couple months, whereas some recommend using them forever. We'll talk about why protein is so important and the differences in the types of protein supplements in an upcoming chapter. But in the meantime, realize that right now you need to think about which protein supplements you'll use after surgery.

Don't try too many brands of protein powder before surgery though. It is common for your taste preferences to change after surgery. What you like before surgery could be, and often is, different after surgery.

I highly recommend using sample packets of protein powder rather than investing in large jars of supplements that you have never tasted. Protein is expensive and there are literally thousands of brands and flavors to choose from. The taste of protein supplements is subjective and you need to spend some time experimenting with the different flavors before you'll find which one is best for you. I had to try four dozen (yes, that's 48!) different protein brands or flavors before I found two or three that tasted good to me. It's a huge game of experimentation, but it's worth it when you finally find your favorites.

There are several companies that sell samples of protein powder — see the Resources section in the back of the book for a list of these companies.

Protein Shake Maker or Blender

A regular old blender — the one I've had for over 15 years — was great for making my protein shakes. Some people love the personal size blenders that make one serving size at a time. Some like the manual method of a plastic drink bottle with a wire blender ball inside or even just a glass and spoon will do the trick too. It doesn't matter which option you choose, but be sure you have a method for making protein drinks and experiment with the different methods to find which fits best into your lifestyle.

Cell phone and calendar alerts

I use the free website MyMedSchedule.com to keep track of all my medication and vitamin needs and schedule dosing times for everything. I can then set up my account to alert me of my dosing times through an email or a text message sent to my cell phone. I highly recommend this website, it's a godsend!

There are other similar applications available for your smartphone or email system. Or you could set regular interval alarms to ring on your cell phone. Many people find that some sort of alarm system helps them stay on track with remembering to take vitamins and also staying on track with an eating/snacking/drinking schedule. Once your vitamin and eating schedule becomes habit, you won't need the alerts, but in the beginning this can be very helpful. Explore some options now, before surgery, so you're ready to implement the alerts afterward.

Find an angel

A Surgery Angel is a friend within the bariatric community who is your point of contact with the rest of the community while you're having surgery. By now you've established friendships in your support groups and online communities and when your surgery date arrives, they will want to be kept updated on how you're doing.

After you're safely out of surgery and resting again in your room at the hospital, a friend or family member who is with you only needs to call one person to give an update — your Surgery Angel. Then the Angel will pass along the good news of your surgery to anyone else who you want her to contact. Some Angels live in the same town as you and will come visit you in the hospital, but some might live many miles or states away and can support you through email and telephone calls. Often your Surgery Angel will become a close friend or mentor as you begin your journey through the WLS experience.

Get your affairs in order

Nobody likes to think about the risks associated with this surgery, but they are real and we must be prepared to face whatever comes to us. The mortality and complication rates are very low for WLS, so I don't mean to scare you with this section. But let's be real for a moment, okay?

You'll want to make sure your will and living will are both updated and in a place your family can access the paperwork in case anything happens to you. Also be sure that all important account numbers, user identification, password and log-in information is readily available in case it is needed. You may also want to leave a list of email addresses or phone numbers of friends you want contacted if something goes wrong. Some people even write letters to their family members and friends to express their thoughts and feelings. No matter what steps you take to prepare for the worse, be sure to discuss your wishes with your family so they know what to do, and how you want to be cared for, in the event of a serious complication.

Before my surgery I was pretty calm. Not nervous at all and mostly just impatient to get it done and over with so I could start my new life. But on the morning of my surgery, in a last moment fit of nervousness, I quickly wrote down my email passwords, bank account numbers and a couple email addresses for friends on a sticky-note and attached it to the top of my laptop computer with the title "just in case." Your list can be just that informal or it can be a more diligent and thoughtful list of information.

Record your weight, measurements and take photos

Start now to keep detailed documentation of your weight, measurements, BMI, and body fat percentage. I created a weight and measurement chart to keep track of my numbers over time. By documenting this information from the very beginning, I have a solid record of my progress over the past several years.

Record your current height, weight and all your measurements in your chart. And if you have access to a body fat percentage device, have that measured too.

The day before your surgery — or the day before you begin a pre-op diet — take a bunch of photos of yourself. Get all angles – front, back, side, close up, full body. You might also want to consider some photos without many clothes — naked or maybe a bathing suit. Not only will these photos be a visual accounting of your weight loss journey and a reminder of how far you've come, but they might also be handy when you're thinking about plastic or reconstructive surgery after you've lost your weight and need to have excess skin removed.

And keep taking pictures! Some people do a monthly series of photos to show the changes in front, back and side profiles. About ten days after my surgery a friend suggested I do a "photo a day" project for a year and put it together in a video when I was done. So I set up my camera on the tripod in my living room and took a picture of my face every morning for the entire first year after my surgery. It's amazing to look back and see the dramatic transformation in myself.

Relax, stay calm, and pamper yourself

It's easy in these last days before surgery to get overly emotional. You're about to embark on a journey to health that is at once terrifying and amazing. Remember to lean on your new friends in the bariatric community — we've all been where you are today and know what you're feeling. Also take time for some self-pampering. Schedule a spa day complete with a relaxing massage, facial, pedicure and manicure or set up a play date with friends for a night on the town with a movie or dancing. Take the time to write your feelings in your WLS journal and record your anxieties, hopes and dreams for the future.

Chapter 3
Life after surgery

Although my actual RNY happened on November 13, 2007, I often have to stop and think about what my actual surgery date was because in my heart, my WLS journey began two weeks before I was on the operating table – October 30, 2007. The surgical process usually begins a number of weeks before your surgery date with a prescribed high-protein, low calorie, liquid diet.

This first month typically happens in three stages.

Two Weeks Before — The specialized diet leading up to your surgery date will be both mentally and physically challenging. But facing those challenges in the weeks before surgery will help the weeks after surgery be easier to handle.

One Week After — The first week after your surgery will be challenging simply because you're healing from a major operation. You're dealing with the physical pain of surgery and emotional challenges of starting a new phase of your life.

Two Weeks After — The second week after surgery is challenging because you're learning a new physical way of eating and starting to establish a new relationship with food while mourning the loss of food as a comfort, companion and celebrant.

The first month or two of surgery is when the most changes happen. It can also be the most overwhelming time as you find your footing and figure out your routines. It's like waking up in a new body and having to learn the basics of life all over again — a "new" body that looks exactly the same, but functions very differently.

Nobody ever said this journey would be easy and during the first few months after surgery you'll probably snarl at anyone who says you took the "easy way out." But the rewards are great and worth every bit of the hard work, sacrifice, and turmoil you'll be confronting. During the first month after my surgery I lost 27 pounds, was finally able to sleep through the night (something I hadn't done in years) and some of my medical issues were beginning to disappear. Even though these first four weeks are hard, there's a lot to celebrate too. Let's take a closer look at each of these three stages.

Two weeks pre-op

Most surgeons now require patients to follow a strict two week high-protein, low calorie liquid diet before surgery. Each bariatric program is different, of course – some require four or six weeks on a pre-op diet and some allow limited solid food (usually vegetables or grilled lean chicken or fish) for one of your daily meals with the remaining being liquid protein drinks; mine was all liquid and lasted two weeks. (Some surgeons don't ask patients to do a pre-op diet, so don't panic if yours doesn't require this step.) No matter the exact content of this pre-operative diet, the reasons behind it are important.

First, this strict diet will help you lose weight before surgery. Any weight you can lose before surgery will make you that much healthier and allow for a safer surgery. A liquid diet that is low in fat and simple carbohydrates will also help to shrink your liver. Your liver is located right in front of your stomach and must be lifted out of the way during surgery.

In morbidly obese patients the liver is often enlarged due to a condition called non-alcoholic fatty liver disease. Fatty Liver tends to develop in people who are overweight or obese or have diabetes, high cholesterol or high triglycerides, and in one study 60% of bariatric surgery patients were found to have this disease.[3]

By losing weight and restricting food intake to a basic high-protein diet, the fat deposits in the liver will be reduced and the liver will be less cumbersome for the surgeon. This will help to reduce the risk of complications or injury to the liver during the surgery.

Second, a pre-op diet will help you lose more weight after your surgery. Yes, that's right. For every 1 percent of your excess body weight you lose before surgery, studies show that you will have a 1.8 percent higher weight loss at 12-months post-op than those who did not lose weight pre-op. Plus, it's been shown that those who lose more than 5 percent of their excess weight will have a shorter operating time by 36 minutes.

Conversely, weight gain before surgery comes with consequences. For every one unit on the BMI scale you increase your weight, you will lose 1.34 percent less weight than those who did not gain pre-op.[4]

From my own personal experience — and the stories of others I've met along the way — I believe that a strict pre-op diet helps us to begin the process of training our mind to eat in a different way and prepares us emotionally for the drastic changes about to come. The emotional journey of WLS is a tough one and getting a jumpstart is an added benefit.

On my pre-op diet, I was limited to three 8-ounce protein shakes, 8-ounces of broth or clear soup, and one fiber drink per day with the addition of 64-ounces of water and other non-calorie fluids. The first four days were brutal and I had more cravings for food than ever before. I cried for the want of food.

I was obsessed with dreaming up recipes in my head and thinking of food every waking moment. Every minute I was home and the television was on, it was tuned to some cooking show or another. I obsessively searched the internet for new recipes or food ideas or just photos of food to drool over. I wasn't sure if I'd make it through a whole two weeks like this. It was an hourly struggle to be faithful to the diet plan and not cheat.

Later I learned that what I was experiencing — obsessive thoughts of food and an obsessive preoccupation with any topic related to food — was normal based on the findings of the Minnesota Starvation Study. This was a scientific experiment conducted during World War II on a group of volunteers who were subjected to severe calorie restriction and their behavior and medical condition studied. The results are enlightening as they relate to the level of starvation we are experiencing with bariatric surgery. I recommend you take the time to read about the study (find a link to the online report in the Resources section).

During my weeks and months of waiting for insurance approval I came across the saying, "I am stronger than myself." This phrase became my mantra in these early days of the pre-op diet and right after my surgery when eating was severely restricted.

I am stronger than that cookie.
I am stronger than that hamburger.
I am stronger than my cravings.
I am stronger than my willpower.
I am stronger than myself.

I played that saying over and over in my mind throughout the day as I faced temptation at every turn. It worked for me. And sometimes, even now, many years post-op, that mantra is still helpful when I'm faced with a craving I don't want to give in to. I'm a strong and powerful woman... but sometimes I need to be stronger than myself.

Something happened on the fifth day of the pre-op diet. I turned a corner – physically and emotionally. Suddenly I realized that I was satisfied with the amount of food I was eating and that I really could survive on such a small amount of calories while still getting the nourishment I needed. There was also a mental shift. The cravings were still there, but somehow I had a peace about my ability to accomplish this difficult task.

Because I was able to face the craving demons before surgery, I believe it made my post-op eating an easier adjustment.

The week of surgery

For most Roux-en-Y patients the hospital stay is two to three days. People who have their surgery done with an open incision (as opposed to laparoscopically) can expect a slightly longer hospital stay.

While in the hospital your surgeon will give you pain medication to minimize any discomfort you may feel. If the pain medication you are given is not working properly or is making you nauseous, be sure to let your doctor know so they can make an adjustment. This happened to me while I was in the hospital. I was given a morphine pump to control my pain, however, the morphine made me sick to my stomach. Believe me, having the dry heaves after an abdominal surgery is not a pleasant experience. But as soon as my pain medication was changed and I was given anti-nausea medicine I was pain-free and comfortable during my hospital stay.

The first day — the day of your surgery — you will likely not be able to eat or drink anything, not even ice chips. This will allow time for your new stomach/pouch to heal. The following morning you will be taken for your "swallow test" to check to see if there are any leaks in your newly formed digestive system. Some surgeons do this the same day as the surgery and some even do it during surgery. Ask your doctor how he handles this process. The swallow test involves swallowing some barium and having x-rays taken of your abdomen. This allows the technician to look at your pouch to ensure everything is stitched up correctly and there are no leaks in the staple lines. The hardest part of this test, for me, was standing upright and still for the several minutes the test takes.

Once you pass this test you'll be given water to sip. Usually it is served in a one-ounce medicine cup and you'll need to sip that water for fifteen minutes – yes, it'll take you the full fifteen minutes to drink one ounce of water. Then you'll refill the cup and start over. Sounds easy, huh? But it's not easy for most people. It's a monumental feat to drink just four ounces of water in an hour. But this is an important training step. It'll help you learn what a "sip" is and how to take your time drinking.

Later that day you may graduate to a larger variety of liquids like gelatin, broth, hot tea or protein shakes. I remained on this liquid diet while in the hospital.

As always, some surgeons have a different protocol and you'll follow whatever your surgeon recommends. I know of some patients who were eating soft, pureed food before leaving the hospital while others got nothing more than water to drink. Each program is different and your surgeon will have very specific reasons for the program that's chosen for their patients.

Once you get home from the hospital you will probably remain on a liquid diet for the rest of the first week – either a clear liquid diet or full liquids. Some programs require patients to remain on a clear liquid diet for the first week of gastric bypass surgery. Some programs allow patients to include "full liquids" such as yogurt, cream soups and pudding.

When I came home from the hospital I was on full liquids and was required to drink three protein shakes in order to take in 60-80 grams of protein per day. I was also required to take in 64 ounces of water each day. Even though it is expected that in the first week or two it will be nearly impossible to meet the water and protein goals - you are expected to try your best during this time. You'll be eating about one to two ounces of food (full liquids) at one setting during this early stage.

As for the recovery of surgery during this first week, I came home from the hospital with a prescription for pain medication. I took one dose the evening I arrive home. After that I didn't need anything stronger than Tylenol. Many people experience the same pain-free recovery that I did. However, we're all different and we will all have different experiences. Many people have harder recoveries and rely on pain medication for a week or two. If you are one who continues to feel pain, then my best advice to you is this: Don't be a hero! Pain is not desirable, so take your pain meds and let your body heal in comfort.

You'll also be very, very tired during these first few days out of the hospital. Sleep as much as you can and let your body recuperate. Keep walking regularly to reduce the risk of blood clots, of course. But if you want to take a couple naps during the day, do it!

Two weeks post-op

I was amazed at how well I felt after the first week of recovery. I was able to get around just fine and was healing quickly. I continued to get tired easily in these first couple weeks and needed at least one daily nap. I was thankful I had taken five weeks off work so I could give my body the time it needed to heal properly.

The eating part of the recovery process was still a challenge. Depending on your surgeon's requirements and nutritionist guidelines, you may continue eating full liquids one week after your WLS — some patients progress to soft foods at this point. No matter what your guidelines, be sure to follow what your doctor's mandates. They have developed your nutritional program based on years of experience and helping thousands of other post-op patients. Your surgeon saw your innards, he knows what he did to your guts and he knows what needs to happen for you to heal properly based on what he did during surgery. Following the rules in these early weeks is literally putting your life in the hands of your medical team — don't deviate from these important rules.

I was on full liquids this second week after surgery until I had my follow-up appointment with my surgeon's office for my two-week post-op appointment. After being checked out to make sure I was healing as expected, I was cleared to begin the next phase of my eating plan which included soft foods such as egg salad, pate`, hummus, refried beans and soft or melted cheese. I was also allowed to add up to one tablespoon of a "side item" which included either soft cooked vegetables or a grain-based food (from a very limited list).

You'll be given guidelines for water and protein right after surgery. Usually you'll be expected to get 64 ounces of water and 60-80 grams of protein per day. Many surgeons or nutritionist forget to tell you that they know you won't be able to get all that in immediately after surgery. Just do the best you can and get as much of both as possible each day. It'll be a full time job to eat and drink and take your vitamins. It'll be overwhelming and you'll wonder why you're the only one who can't do it. But we all struggled with this. The best we can do is just our best. Do a little bit better tomorrow and a bit better than that the next day. It's a process that you have to work at.

Also remember that the number one reason patients end up back in the hospital after WLS is due to dehydration. Some signs to watch for with dehydration include dry mouth, excessive thirst, weakness and fatigue, headaches, rapid heartbeat, nausea, muscle cramps, rapid breathing and dizziness. If you think you might be dehydrated, call your surgeon for assistance.

Other people who have gone through this journey before me kept saying that the first month is the hardest part of the whole surgery process — and that's true (until you hit the maintenance phase, but we won't get into that just yet). Once you pass the six-week mark, things get easier and the variety of food you're allowed is much greater. So hold on during these first weeks and know it's going to get better soon.

The craziness that ensues

No matter how much research you do or how fully you believe you understand what life will be like after weight loss surgery, you are going to be experiencing a lot of crazy stuff you never expected. Or maybe you expected it, but didn't realize how crazy the crazy really gets. This section is my attempt to warn you that it's coming and hopefully bring you some assurance that you aren't losing your mind.

You will experience extreme mood swings, crying jags and bouts of depression followed by a feeling of being overjoyed at the tiniest hurdle you jump. Your body will do strange things, your emotions will be all over the map and your hair might even start to shed. And all these unusual things will happen at the exact same time that you're making major life-altering changes to your relationship with food, your eating plan, and the way you exercise. It can all be very overwhelming. But there is a light at the end of the tunnel.

Let's look at why there's so much "craziness" in these first few months after surgery... there really is a scientific reason why.

Hormones are raging

An average adult has 30 billion fat cells with a weight of 30 lbs. If excess weight is gained as an adult, fat cells increase in size about fourfold before dividing to create more fat cells.[5] Fat cells aren't just tiny storage vessels for excess energy; inside each cell you'll find a little factory that produces all sorts of fun stuff. In fact, scientists are now referring to fat cells as part of the endocrine system because they can release hormones straight into the bloodstream — just like the thyroid and pituitary glands. One of the main hormones produced in fat cells is estrogen, present in both men and women. (Yes men, you also have estrogen, so don't ignore this important section!)

As we lose weight all those excess hormones are released from the fat cells and begin roaming the streets of our circulatory system, looking for trouble. Estrogen is the new street thug of weight loss. And we women know what excess estrogen can do, right? Can we say premenstrual syndrome?

Estrogen dominance comes with some very serious side effects including mood swings, depression, irritability, dry skin and hair, insomnia, fatigue, fuzzy thinking, low libido and a general feeling of PMS-like symptoms. Women may also experience unexpected menstruation cycles at unscheduled times or those who haven't had a regular cycle in years may suddenly have a period shortly after surgery (or before if you're losing weight on a pre-op diet). It is common to have these types of feelings and physical symptoms for several months during the rapid weight loss phase of post-surgery life.

It might be a good idea to warn your family of the impending craziness so they don't lock you in a closet for your moodiness. The good news is that it's a direct result of losing weight, so celebrate the fact that your surgery is working and everything is going according to plan. Also rest assured that this isn't a permanent condition. Once your weight loss stabilizes or slows down a bit, the hormone craziness goes away.

You don't have to endure this hormonal surge on your own. Many people find that the emotional upheaval is just too much to bear and require some medication to take the edge off. Talk to your surgeon or PCP about your options for anti-depressant medication or other options to help you through this difficult time.

The bariatric community can be a valuable resource during these times. If you're experiencing something you think is strange or abnormal, asking a fellow bariatric patient about their experiences can help you determine if you're within the norm or if you need to seek medical attention. We've all been where you are, lean on us for support.

Hair loss & shedding

Yes, you'll most likely lose some hair after weight loss surgery. It's normal and it's okay. The biological word for hair loss typically experienced after any traumatic event is Telogen effluvium. This type of thinning or shedding of hair after an emotionally or physically traumatic event is temporary and indicates that the hair follicles have prematurely entered the "resting stage" of the normal grown cycle. The hair loss is related to the trauma of your weight loss surgery, the emotional divorce from food, and the extreme reduction in caloric intake. Nothing you do can reverse the hair loss or make it stop before it's done shedding. No amount of extra protein, vitamins, shampoos or supplements can stop the shedding and nothing can speed up the regrowth. You just have to wait for it to run its course and be patient.

Registered dietitian, David Kellenberger, MPAS, RD, PA-C, explains the hair loss cycle after bariatric surgery below:

> *"Human hair has a two stage growth cycle. The growth phase is called anagen and 90% of our hair follicles are in this phase at any given time. The resting phase is called telogen. About 5-15% of your hair is in the resting phase at any given time. Telogen effluvium has to do with stress to the body and hormonal changes that can occur and causes more hair follicles to enter the resting phase. The hair in the resting phase at the time of surgery is most likely the hair you will shed which happens when new hair grows and old hair is released – usually about 3 to 4 months after surgery."* (source: drdkim.net)

Read some more …

Yes, I know I seem to be a broken record about this whole reading thing. But I'm going to point out that book recommendation again because I think it contains such essential information for us after weight loss surgery. So, if you haven't gotten it already, get the *Emotional First Aid Kit: A practical guide for life after bariatric surgery* by Cynthia Alexander.

It's one of those books that you can't read straight through. It's a small book but it's packed full of emotional assistance for post-op patients and you can only read small bits of it at a time. It took me six months to read it my first time. But it's a tremendous help for any weight loss surgery patient struggling with the emotional craziness that happens after surgery.

Being active

Many people ask how soon after surgery should they start exercising. The answer? About three hours.

Right after your surgery the nurses will start bugging you about getting up and walking. Walk, walk, walk! The purpose of this early exercise is all about preventing the formation of blood clots and causing serious complications.

The instructions I received where: "Walk for 5 minutes every hour that you're awake." So I was up and walking around the day of my surgery just like you will be. In the early days after surgery my walking was very slow and a lot of hard work. I used the treadmill in the weeks after my surgery and I was lucky to hit a speed of 2 miles per hour for that full 5 minutes. And this is coming from a patient who was walking 60-90 minutes at a brisk pace several days a week before surgery. So expect to have a slow start when you're recovering. The more I worked at it, the easier it got.

Not only is this early walking good for avoiding blood clots, but it's also an excellent way to begin a new habit of exercise. Walking is a great way to keep your body active and get in shape. Some people don't do any other form of exercise after WLS — walking is enough for many.

Once you get home from the hospital, walking remains essential. The "five minutes every hour" rule is a good one to implement - remember that the blood clot risk continues for several weeks after surgery. Eventually you'll incorporate a formal exercise routine which might be more walking or other forms of activity like aerobics, bicycling, swimming or weight training. Check with your surgeon to find out when you're cleared for activities more strenuous than walking, though. In the early days after surgery, your goal needs to be: "Just do a little bit more tomorrow."

Living Your Post-op Life

Once you progress to normal foods around the six-week mark and you're cleared for exercise, it's time to settle into your post-op life routine.

I know it seems unbelievable that this chapter is only 10 pages long and it's supposed to cover all the physical parts of the WLS life. But I guess that's my point in this chapter being so concise. The physical part of this journey is the easy part.

I've said it hundreds to time - and will continue to say it hundreds more — the physical surgery is only about 10% of this process. The other 90% is all about getting your head screwed on straight; developing a healthy relationship with food; learning to live a new kind of life and figuring out how to mold your life in such a way that the weight loss will be a lifelong success. The mental part of this journey is where the real hard work happens.

Chapter 4
Your altered body

Before I had RNY I did all the typical research and reading about how the surgery works and what the surgeon does to make my stomach smaller and reroute my digestive tract. I attended a couple different comprehensive seminars held by my surgeon's office that explained how the surgery works and what it all meant to my nutrition and health for the long term. I attended a support group for over a year before my surgery and read online forums for nearly 18 months. I understood all the details of surgery and what was going to be done to my body.

But it was only after I started doing research about the human digestive system, nutrition, and metabolism and how it all works together; that I was more fully able to appreciate why Roux-en-Y works. I didn't pay very close attention in biology class when I was in school and the stuff that I did learn, I'd forgotten in the 25 years since I sat in Mrs. Currie's class. Since I started my digging into WLS, I have done more reading and research on the human body than I ever did in the all years I sat in a classroom.

With this more in-depth understanding, I'm better able to understand my body and adjust my behaviors based on what it requires now that it's been altered. Once you begin asking the questions how your altered body works, you begin by asking questions about basic biology and how things work differently now.

Some common questions might be: What size is my stomach pouch and will it stretch? How does malabsorption work? And how long does it last? What happens to food after I eat it and where are the nutrients absorbed? And a thousand more questions. Ask them all and dig into the research until you have your answers — and keep digging even after you have a good understanding. Doctors and scientists are learning new things everyday about how our bodies work and we can continue to learn how those new discoveries apply to weight loss surgery. Knowledge is power and the more you know and understand about how your body works — before and after surgery — the better chance you have at long term success with WLS.

So let's answer some of the basic questions about how the body works. Welcome to Biology 101! We'll look at what the body looked like before surgery and what it's like now that it's been altered.

The Stomach

The average human stomach can hold up to one to four liters of food and fluid at a time, that's around four to sixteen cups!.[6] At rest your stomach is about the size of a man's fist but when filled with food and liquid it can expand to the size of a football. Your stomach is a powerful muscle with a vast network of nerves all along the interior tissue. Digestive enzymes and hydrochloric acid (known as gastric acid) is produced in the cells of the mucus lining of the stomach to aid in digestion. The stomach's primary function is to churn food and mix it with gastric acid so it is prepared for the small intestines where absorption takes place.

The Gastric Pouch

Your new RNY pouch, at the time of surgery, is about one ounce in size and can hold about two or three ounces of food. (Of course, each pouch size will be different based on individual surgical techniques, but the one-ounce size seems to be most common). Your surgeon made your pouch out of the least-stretchy part of your stomach - the cardia – which means that your pouch will expand to accommodate food, but it is difficult to "stretch out" permanently unless you abuse it. The actual act of pouch expansion when we eat is what gives us the physical sensation of fullness or satisfaction after a meal.

Even though the pouch is difficult to stretch, that doesn't mean it stays the same size forever. Your body is pretty smart and as soon as it figures out you've rearranged things, it immediately begins to fix itself. The process is called Intestinal Adaptation and has been studied extensively in patients who have various forms of intestinal diseases and cancers which might require a portion of their stomach or bowel be removed. But their research helps us understand more about how our bodies work after WLS.

Your pouches will grow over time as part of the adaptation process. A mature pouch is about six to nine ounces in size and can naturally expand to hold

Where are nutrients absorbed in the small intestine?[8]

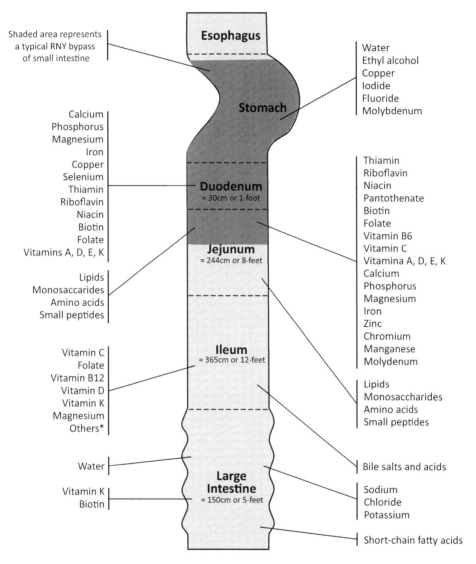

Shaded area represents a typical RNY bypass of small intestine

Esophagus

Stomach

Water
Ethyl alcohol
Copper
Iodide
Fluoride
Molybdenum

Calcium
Phosphorus
Magnesium
Iron
Copper
Selenium
Thiamin
Riboflavin
Niacin
Biotin
Folate
Vitamins A, D, E, K

Duodenum
≈ 30cm or 1-foot

Thiamin
Riboflavin
Niacin
Pantothenate
Biotin
Folate
Vitamin B6
Vitamin C
Vitamina A, D, E, K
Calcium
Phosphorus
Magnesium
Iron
Zinc
Chromium
Manganese
Molydenum

Jejunum
≈ 244cm or 8-feet

Lipids
Monosaccarides
Amino acids
Small peptides

Vitamin C
Folate
Vitamin B12
Vitamin D
Vitamin K
Magnesium
Others*

Ileum
≈ 365cm or 12-feet

Lipids
Monosaccarides
Amino acids
Small peptides

Water

Bile salts and acids

Vitamin K
Biotin

Large Intestine
≈ 150cm or 5-feet

Sodium
Chloride
Potassium

Short-chain fatty acids

*Many additional nutrients may be absorbed from the ileum depending on transit time.

Reprinted with permission from Cengage Learning Nelson Education as published in Advanced Nutrition and Human Metabolism by Grooper & Smith (copyright 2009).

about eight to twelve ounces of food at a time. A pouch reaches maturity at about two years post-op. But this growth process begins immediately after surgery and by six months post-op your pouch has grown to about two-thirds of its maturity level. Once you are a year post op your pouch is no longer the same one-ounce it was at the time of your surgery, it's more like three or four ounces and can hold five to seven ounces of food.

Studies have shown that the size of your pouch has very little to do with your overall success with weight loss. Your success has more to do with how well you follow your eating and exercise plan and how well you follow the rules of the pouch.[7] Success depends on changing the way you live your life and the behavioral changes you make in the way you eat and think about food.

The Small Intestine

Along with a smaller stomach pouch which only holds a small amount of food, RNY also involves bypassing a portion of your small intestine. Your small intestine is divided into three distinct sections and each section has its own job assignment with the primary function being digestion of the food we eat and the absorption of nutrients from food and supplements.

The small intestine is almost exclusively responsible for absorbing all nutrients from the food we eat. This includes **micro**nutrients (vitamins and minerals) as well as **macro**nutrients (protein, fat, carbohydrates = calories). These two types of nutrients are absorbed differently, so we'll discuss both.

The small intestine is not merely a hollow tube that food rides along until it exits the body. There's a lot of action going on inside the pipeline. The intestinal tract contains strong muscles that contract in a circular and longitudinal motion to propel food along the system. Digestive enzymes are produced in the small intestine and mixed with the food as it's churned with these muscle contractions. All along the inside of the small intestine there is a brush border which is made up of finger-like tentacles, called villi, that project out into the hollow tube of the intestinal tract. The villi is responsible for grabbing nutrients from food that passes by and then sending those nutrients into the body.

Think of villi as tiny little factory workers in a manufacturing plant. Food is moved down the assembly line (small intestine) and workers (villi) grab nutrients from the food. The workers then process it for use within the body's cells. Each villi crew is responsible for very specific tasks when it comes to micro-nutrient absorption. Some nutrients are so important that the body has set up several absorption points along the small intestine while others only have one absorption point. Notice the diagram on page 41 to understand where various micro-nutrients are absorbed.

A typical RNY bypass length is about 75 to 150 centimeters or about 2½ to 5 feet. Each surgeon has their own method to determine the bypass length, ask your doctor about your specific surgery.

When a portion of your small intestine is bypassed for weight loss surgery your body is not able replace those absorption points somewhere else along the intestinal tract. Once that little nutrient manufacturing plant is gone, it's gone forever. When you eat food containing those vitamins and minerals, your body is no longer able to grab nutrients from the food because the food will never pass by those points again. As noted in the diagram, there might be some residual absorption in the lower part of the intestinal tract depending on transit time, but there's no guarantee of that additional absorption.

For example, look at the diagram and notice there are two absorption points for calcium - before surgery when you would drink milk, the duodenum and jejunum would recognize the calcium in the milk and grab the nutrient as milk passed by. But now the milk you drink will never pass those two spots again because of the bypass portion of your surgery. Therefore, it is impossible for your body to grab calcium from the milk you drink - or any other food that is high in calcium. There may be some passive absorption in other parts of the intestine, but science hasn't yet determined the effectiveness of passive absorption. So the only way you can get calcium in your diet is to take a calcium supplement.

A supplement is developed by extracting the nutrient from food and preparing it in such a way that your body is ready to use it without first having the extract the nutrient using the villi brush border system. It's important to know what other vitamins and minerals are no longer absorbed because of your bypassed small intestine. We'll discuss nutrients in more depth in Chapter 6 and 7.

Intestinal Adaptation

Your body immediately begins to compensate for the surgery. Once your body realizes that your stomach is now the size of a walnut, a portion of your intestine has been bypassed and you aren't absorbing all the calories you're eating, it begins to figure out how to become more efficient. This is called Intestinal Adaptation.[9]

Your intestines grow wider (increased diameter) and also increased the effectiveness of villi along the intestinal wall so your body is better able to grab macronutrients (protein, fat, carbs) and calories as food passes by. The villi becomes longer and stronger than it was before the bypass so the shortened length of your small intestine becomes highly efficient at doing the work of the portion that's no longer there for macronutrient absorption.

This adaptation process takes a while to happen. Even though adaption begins immediately (as soon as four days post-op), the entire process takes about two to three years to complete. By three years post-op you're likely absorbing every single calorie you eat.

Don't confuse micro-nutrient absorption with macronutrient absorption, though. Micronutrients (vitamins and minerals) are only absorbed at their specifically assigned locations. Macronutrient absorption (protein, fat, carbohydrates) happens all along the digestive tract and is not dependent upon certain areas of the small intestine.

Villi is not the only part of your anatomy that adapts though. Your pouch will grow over time as well. It starts out as a one ounce sized stomach but will eventually expand and grow to maturity of about 6 to 9 ounces in size (and able to hold about 8 to 12 ounces of food). This is normal and natural and nothing to panic about. This natural growth is part of your body's way of keeping you alive and healthy because you simply can't survive on a stomach that remains one ounce. The stomach is a living organ within your body, so growth is natural.

Even though our body adapts to the surgery to over time and our eating patterns change in the few years following surgery, I firmly believe the tool continues to work for the rest of our lives. As long as we protect it and be kind to it to avoid over-stretching a mature pouch and as long as we eat the right foods and take our supplements. By understanding that it grows, matures and changes over time you also understand that you have to adapt your behavior to what's going on inside your body, you can remain successful in your weight loss for the rest of your life.

What is Dumping Syndrome?

I don't dump. Sorta, kinda. Well, I do dump, but I have a pretty high threshold for sugar before I get that awful feeling of death known as dumping syndrome. But because I have such a high threshold, I technically consider myself a non-dumper. And yes, I've pushed that sugar limit further than I should have on occasion and I'll tell you more about that later. First, let's understand what dumping syndrome is and what goes on inside your body when you're dumping.

Dumping Syndrome is a medical term used to describe a series of events that happen when stomach contents are literally "dumped" rapidly into the small intestine. It is usually triggered by too much sugar or fat in food. Dumping symptoms aren't fun: nausea, cramping, weakness, sweating, faintness, and diarrhea, but let's break it down into steps.

You eat some type of food with too much sugar or too much fat – it's the content of the food that is the trigger for dumping, not the texture or consistency of the food.

In a normal stomach (before surgery) simple carbohydrates like refined sugar are broken down inside the stomach with enzymes designed specifically for that task. But after surgery you no longer have a normal stomach and because you have no pyloric valve to keep food in the stomach pouch until it's been broken down with gastric acid or enzymes, these foods are emptied from the pouch into the small intestines fairly quickly.

Once this food reaches the intestines, the body is unable to break down the sugar/fat so it tries to get rid of the offending food as quickly as possible. The body literally goes into panic mode.

Fluid from all over the body is rushed to the intestines to help flush the food out – this causes intestinal cramping and a bloated feeling.

The body is in panicked survival mode or fight-or-flight mode, so it releases endorphins to help ensure its survival — this causes rapid heartbeat and sometimes increased blood pressure and often sweating or an overheated feeling.

The body realizes there's too much sugar in the system — this will show as a spike in your blood glucose levels. Because of these elevated blood glucose levels, the body then releases extra insulin to help "soak up" some of that sugar and process it as quickly as possible — this will often show as a dramatic drop in blood glucose levels and may result in a hypoglycemic reaction.

As a result of the excess fluid in the intestinal tract and the body's all-out effort to rid itself of the offending food, you'll often end up with diarrhea or an urgent need to use the bathroom. Some people also report an excess amount of urination after a dumping episode.

Each person is different when it comes to dumping. The above scenario outlines the typical biological reactions of dumping syndrome — but any one of those steps might be skipped or intensified in each different person who dumps. For some people dumping will last 20 minutes and they instantly feel better. Some people suffer for hours or even days. I have a friend who proclaims she's a three-day-dumper as it takes her body a full three days to get back to normal afterward. We're all different and each one of us won't know what dumping is like until we actually experience it for ourselves.

The ASMBS reports that about 85% of RNY patients will experience dumping syndrome at some time after surgery.[10] But that high number includes all instances of dumping, so even if a person only dumps one time after surgery, they are included in that percentage.

A more realistic statistic is reported in an article by a group of gastroenterologists who study various types of intestinal bypass.[11] About 41% of patients experience regular dumping syndrome and that percentage includes all dumpers of sugar and fat combined. Only about 1-5% of patients experience severe dumping symptoms that can be classified as disabling.

As I mentioned earlier, I consider myself part of the 59% of patients who do not dump. However, because I do experience dumping symptoms if I push my limits too far, I am technically a dumper.

My threshold is about 40 grams sugar before I start to feel the effects. That's a package of peanut M&M's or a whole slice of cake. Yes, I've eaten both of those things on rare occasions … in fact I live my life and plan my food as if I were a dumper and limit my intake to the recommended 10 grams sugar per meal. I'm perfectly satisfied with three bites of birthday cake and my chocolate craving is easily quenched with a chocolate protein shake, protein hot cocoa, or a couple Hershey's Kisses.

Some people don't have a problem with sugar but dump on too much fat and vice versa. Many people who don't experience physical symptoms may actually be experiencing medical symptoms, such as increased blood glucose levels, and not even realize it. I know many people who have a limit of 5 grams of sugar but more commonly the standard limit is "single digits of sugar" — so 9 grams or less is a good rule of thumb.

Within the medical community dumping syndrome is considered an undesirable side effect of Roux-en-Y. However, psychologists and bariatric professionals know that dumping syndrome can be an effective behavior modification tool for patients who need a method for managing an uncontrollable sweet-tooth. Even for those patients who are non-dumpers, like me, the fear of dumping is enough to keep us from overindulging in foods we shouldn't.

My Body Talks to Me

Isn't it wonderful how our bodies will figure out a way to send us a signal when it wants (or doesn't want) something? Because we've had our anatomy rearranged with WLS, the signals we received before surgery might not be the same signals we'll receive after surgery.

For instance, your new stomach pouch will behave drastically different than your original full-sized stomach when it comes to hunger and satiety.

The stomach has a vast network of nerves — both large and small — that send signals to your brain to let you know when you're full or hungry. But during Roux-en-Y surgery the nerves in your stomach are damaged when the surgeon creates your new stomach pouch. It takes several months for those nerves to repair themselves and start working again. For some, those nerves begin working again in just two or three months. For others, it might take a year or two. Some people will get the feeling back but never have "full signal strength" again while others will have ravenous hunger just like before surgery. We're all different, so you'll discover what your body does when it happens.

During these early weeks and months after surgery we'll often experience what we think of as hunger. But most likely it is a psychological signal rather than true hunger pangs. This is referred to as Head Hunger. Tracy, a support leader from Barix Clinic, defines head hunger as "that thing that makes you think you want to eat even when you're already full or should be full."[12] Our brain is pretty smart and knows how to make its cravings and desires look and feel like real hunger. It takes practice to separate real physical hunger from psychological head hunger, but it is possible, but know that it'll be an ongoing battle we'll need to face for a lifetime.

Your body changes a lot after surgery. And with those changes, it needs to find new ways to communicate with you so you'll understand what it needs. You just need to pay attention and listen to what it's telling you.

I personally never feel hunger like I did before surgery — that gnawing, rumbling feeling in the pit of your stomach. It's refreshing not to have that overwhelming feeling anymore. But when my body needs food it lets me know.

My new hunger signal: light-headedness, slight headache, an "empty" feeling and a general intellectual knowledge that I need food.

My new full signal: a cross between a hiccup and a burp - a tiny, quiet, rumbling mini-hiccup that nobody notices but me and also an intellectual knowledge that I should not eat another bite.

Other WLS patients report several different types of full signals. Sneezes, runny noses or hiccups or burps are some other common signals.

After gastric bypass surgery it is very important to drink 64 ounces of water every day. Water is normally absorbed in the stomach — and since most of your stomach is bypassed now, you need to be sure that you get in all your water every day so that the rest of your digestive tract has the chance to do the job the stomach used to do. We know that once we feel actual "thirst" that it's too late — we've already entered the beginning stages of dehydration. When we wake up in the morning, we're often already dehydrated, so it's important to drink first thing in the morning. If I neglect drinking enough water, my body tells me about it.

My new "must drink" signal: my ears plug up — like what happens when you're on an airplane. Until I drink about 20 ounces of water in the morning my left ear will be clogged up, finally mid-morning it'll pop and all is right with the world again.

So the lesson here is that we have to pay very close attention to our bodies. Once you are in-tune with the subtle signals of communication that your body is telling you, these overwhelming lifestyle changes of eating and drinking and taking vitamins become routine and are ingrained in your daily lives.

Chapter 5
The rules have a reason

After weight loss surgery we are given many new and unusual rules that we must abide by for the rest of our lives. But the idea that we must change the way we think about any one behavior forever can be daunting. So when we're faced with a whole list of new rules — and behavior changes — the change might feel overwhelming. So overwhelming we're tempted to not follow the rules at all.

Personally I'm a bit of a rebel and unless I know exactly why I must follow a rule and understand the reason behind that rule - I will most likely find a way around it. It reminds me of a line in the song by Jason Gray: "*Give me rules, I will break them. Show me lines, I will cross them.*" But understanding why the rule exists helps us to be more compliant with these new rules.

Rule 1: No Drinking With Meals

No drinking with meals or for 30 to 60 minutes after a meal (this includes snacks too). Let's explore the reasons why this rule is so important and what happens when we don't follow the rule.

The Old Anatomy

As we discussed briefly in the previous chapter, after Roux-en-Y you no longer have the same stomach anatomy as you did before surgery. In a normal stomach there is the pyloric valve between the stomach and small intestine to keep food inside the stomach while it begins the digestive process.

The stomach is a powerful muscle that contracts around the food in a churning motion. The stomach releases gastric acid (made up mostly of hydrochloric acid and various enzymes) to further break down food as it's churned. As food is broken down into a liquid the pyloric valve (a trap door, really) opens to let some food particles out of the stomach and into the small intestine for absorption. This churning process continues and the pyloric valve will keep opening and closing as more food is prepared for release. This process can take two to three hours in a normal stomach. It's much different after Roux-en-Y gastric bypass surgery.

The New Anatomy

After RNY the pyloric valve is no longer part of the newly formed gastric pouch. It remains at the bottom of the stomach which is bypassed, so we will never use the pylorus again to control the flow of food from the pouch to the small intestine.

Your new stomach pouch now functions as a funnel — a larger bowl shape at the top with a small narrow opening at the bottom. The food you eat is held in place in the larger upper portion of the funnel and gravity (and some minor muscle contractions and churning) allows food to slowly flow out the lower narrow opening at the bottom of the pouch. That narrow opening is called the anastomosis or "stoma" for short.

With your new pouch you must now mimic the action of the pyloric valve manually and the only way to keep food in your pouch is to eat dense foods and not mix it with liquid.

The Food

The more dense the food, the longer it can stay in the pouch. The softer and more liquid the food, the sooner it will empty from the pouch. Dense food can stay in your pouch for ninety minutes to two hours if you don't drink water. But the moment you add water (or any liquid) to the pouch, you are creating a "soup" that will quickly empty out of your pouch.

Soft foods that slide straight through the stomach pouch are called "slider foods" and include things like yogurt, soup, pudding or cottage cheese. Although these may be good foods to consume in the early stages after surgery, be careful not to get into the habit of using slider foods as your main food source.

Of course when your pouch is empty you'll get hungry sooner. For new post-ops, this isn't a major concern because the hunger hasn't returned fully. But for those further out from surgery, the hunger can be ravenous for some and the primary way to stave off hunger is to keep food in the stomach pouch for as long as possible. This is why it's recommended that the further out you are from surgery, the longer you wait to begin drinking after meals (60-90 minutes).

The New Digestive Process

About 40% of the digestive enzymes required to fully break down simple starch-based carbohydrates is contained in our saliva (known as ptyalin). To break down complex carbohydrates, protein and fat, your body requires the addition of gastric acid and other digestive enzymes normally produced in the stomach. But your new stomach pouch does not produce (in any significant amount) gastric acid or enzymes. This is one of the main reasons why you need to chew, chew, chew really well.

Once food gets to the pouch, the digestive enzymes from your saliva and the limited amount produced by the remaining portion of the stomach go to work on the food to begin breaking it down. Your pouch doesn't churn as much as your old stomach used to, but there is still some movement with that well-chewed food.

The longer food stays in the pouch, the more it is broken down and prepared for the intestines to do their work of grabbing micro- and macro-nutrients from the food. If you wash the food out too quickly a few different things happen. First, if food is not properly prepared for optimal absorption (chewed well, mixed with enzymes) you risk having food move too quickly through your digestive track without the benefit of full nutrient absorption. Second, if food is not well chewed or broken down, you are also at greater risk for intestinal blockages or constipation.

Also realize that if you are washing food out of your pouch while drinking liquid during a meal that you'll be able to eat more food, taking in more calories. The goal of WLS is to eat small portions at meals, but if you are continually emptying your pouch of food during a meal, you'll obviously be able to eat more than your small pouch was designed to hold in one sitting. This habit can lead to weight regain.

The Other Big Risk

There's also the risk of stretching the stoma (the opening between the pouch and intestines). If you have dense food that has not yet begun to be digested in the pouch and you drink water you are forcing dense food through the stoma prematurely. The opening is only about the size of a woman's index finger, but if you habitually push food through the opening before its ready to go, you'll eventually stretch the stoma. This is far more worrisome than stretching your pouch. Once the stoma is stretched it can become the same diameter as the pouch itself. This would essentially create one big long tube that food can be packed into at meals. Need a visual? Stretching your stoma would essentially give you a 20-foot long stomach.

This rule is about biology and medical science because now you need to manually do the work of the pyloric valve that has been bypassed. By following this rule for the rest of your life, you'll properly prepare your food to give your body the best chance of absorbing the vital nutrients it needs for survival as well as achieve the level of satiety needed to reduce hunger between meals.

Tips & Tricks for Rule 1

- Be sure you're well hydrated before meals to avoid excessive thirst afterward.
- During meals, simply don't have a glass of water at your plate.
- To cleanse your palette after a meal, eat 2 grapes for dessert
- Brush your teeth after a meal.
- Look at the clock after the meal to calculate what time you can drink again.
- Use gum or mints to keep your mouth occupied and your mind off drinking.
- Be patient with yourself as you learn, this is a hard rule, it takes practice.

Rule 2: Eat protein first

Eat protein first for each meal or snack. This rule is backed by a few very important reasons — all of which are essential to your good health.

Protein, a macronutrient, is the building block of all cells in your body. What does it mean when they say protein is the "building blocks" for cells? In the simplest of explanations - when your body needs to create new cells, or repair damaged cells, it relies on protein as the primary architecture for those cells. Especially in the weeks after your weight loss surgery, your body is in hyper-repair mode — building new cells and repairing the wounds of surgery. As with any type of surgery, increased protein intake is necessary for proper — and speedy — recovery.

We know we need protein to help repair the damage of surgery, but we also need adequate protein to reduce the risk of muscle wasting during rapid weight loss.

It is known that with any type of weight loss the body is prone to lose a certain percentage of lean muscle mass. Because you are carrying less weight, which requires less strength, the body seems to think this muscle mass may not be needed. But you want to keep it! Muscle is a good thing. Muscle rocks!

Muscle burns more calories at rest than fat does — a pound of muscle will burn about 6 calories per day, whereas a pound of fat will only burn about 2 calories per day. So the more muscle mass we have the greater our calorie burning capacity.

It is recommended that we maintain, or increase, the amount of protein we take in to the same level we did before we started the calorie restricted diet. This means we can decrease all other nutrients, but not protein. Remember, muscle make up 40% of your total body protein and if you don't eat enough protein, the body turns to its own muscle mass to get the protein it needs. By giving your body adequate protein while on a severely restricted calorie intake diet, we are ensuring that we give the body the protein it needs to function without turning to our stored protein (muscle) for those protein requirements.

However, just because the rules say "Protein First" doesn't translate to "Protein Only." A good rule of thumb is: Two bites of protein and one bite of something else. That something else should be veggies, fruit, whole grains or other nutrient-packed food sources.

Rules 3: Drink 64 ounces of water every day

Sip, sip, sip! We hear this mantra all the time (along with walk, walk, walk! and chew, chew, chew!) but do we really realize how important water is for WLS patients?

The daily recommended fluid intake for all adults is around 64-76 ounces per day. The body's total weight is made up of about 60% water and we use water in nearly all functions of daily life including organ function. About 45 ounces is normally lost in urine each day, 4 ounces evaporates in sweat and 8 ounces is lost in feces. The remaining fluid is lost in various ways including evaporation from breathing and other unnoticed ways.

The primary points of absorption of water in the human body are the stomach and the large intestine. Water is absorbed all along the digestive tract, but these two spots are the preferred areas for water to enter the body's cells. But now that your stomach has been bypassed and the new gastric pouch is like a funnel that whisks liquid straight through without staying in the pouch, so the absorption point of the stomach is no longer viable after RNY.

The second absorption point — the large intestine — is pretty far down in the digestive tract and by the time water reaches this point it won't be in the body for very long. So the rest of our digestive tract has to work extra hard to make up for the work the stomach is no longer doing. Therefore, the 64 ounce requirement should be our minimum goal.

But also remember that because you are taking in extra protein in our diets, you need adequate water intake to help the kidneys process this extra nutrient load. The breakdown of protein creates the by product of uric acid which the body must eliminate through the kidneys. If you don't get enough water in your daily diet, these toxins can build up in your body. Excess uric acid can lead to many unwanted medical conditions including gout, diabetes, metabolic syndrome and kidney stones. To stay healthy you must flush your system with lots of fluids.

As we burn fat for energy, the byproducts of this furnace effect is water and carbon dioxide. The water is released from the body through urine and the carbon dioxide is released through your breath. So as you lose fat, your body will naturally produce extra water, but that doesn't remove the requirement for drinking at least 64 ounces of water per day.

Rule 4: No NSAIDs

NSAIDs are non-steroid anti-inflammatory drugs. We know them as Motrin, Excederin, Pepto Bismol, aspirin or any other similar medication — and now we're no longer allowed to use them. But why?

To understand why we can't take NSAIDs we must first understand a bit about the anatomy of the digestive system, specifically the mucosal lining. The mucosal lining is a thin layer (1mm thick) that extends from the mouth all the way through the entire digestive tract — stomach, small intestine and large intestine. This thin membrane protects the delicate flesh of your organs from the harsh chemicals that break down food — hydrochloric acid and gastric acid. Have you ever wondered how your body can break down a T-bone steak into liquid form, but it those same chemicals don't harm your own stomach? It's the mucous membrane's job to protect you from yourself.

NSAIDs work in the body by blocking the production of certain enzymes in the body — Cox-1 and Cox-2. These enzymes, in turn, produce chemicals that cause pain and swelling — prostaglandins. But by blocking the production of those the enzymes, the body is essentially unable to produce the pain-causing chemicals, prostaglandins, and able to eliminate the pain you experience.

Sounds great, right? No, not really. The problem is that not all prostaglandins are created equally and some are actually good to have around. One type of prostaglandin helps to protect the mucosal lining of the stomach and digestive system. So eliminating all prostaglandins from your body will put your mucous lining at risk by causing the layer to become thin and less protective against harsh gastric acid.

NSAIDs are systemic in nature. This means that the pill isn't just dangerous to the areas of the stomach (or pouch) that it touches directly; it will actually work within the body's entire system to reduce prostaglandin production. So you run the risk of compromising the strength of the mucous membrane wherever it happens to be - whether it's in the gastric pouch, small intestine or the bypasses remnant stomach.

What happens when the mucous membrane is thin and gastric acid is able to get through to the tender flesh of your stomach or digestive organs? Ulcers! What's most worrisome is the possibility of developing ulcers in the remnant stomach. The bypassed stomach still produces gastric acid and if the mucosal lining is compromised, you run risk of developing ulcers and all the complications that follow. The problem is that the bypassed stomach - also referred to as the "blind stomach" — cannot be seen. There are no tools that can be put down a patient's throat that can wind its way back up and around to see what's going on inside the bypassed stomach. The only way to know if there is damage in that organ is through surgery.

Those who have battled ulcers will tell you it's no fun at all and a pretty miserable way to live each day. Don't risk it! Just assume that NSAIDs are off limits for the rest of your life and find an alternative treatment for your minor aches and pains. This includes pills you swallow, creams you rub onto skin, patches, nasal sprays or any other medication that contains NSAIDs.

There are some doctors who will allow limited dosing of NSAIDs for patients on a case-by-case basis. Usually it's only allowed after all other alternatives have been tried and only when specific precautions have been taken to reduce the risk of ulcers. Speak to your doctor about the risks so you can weigh the risks against the benefits of using NSAIDs for your special circumstances.

Rule 5: Exercise is a rule

In 2007 the American College of Sports Medicine and the American Heart Association issued guidelines for exercise to lose weight — 60 to 90 minutes of physical activity most days of the week. But why do we need to exercise? Can't the surgery just do the work for us? The weight is just going to melt off anyway, right?

You're probably wondering why exercise is even listed as a rule that needs to be explained. It seems pretty obvious. You exercise so you can lose weight faster, right? Wrong! OK, maybe not completely wrong, but it's sorta-kinda wrong.

Exercise will definitely help you to burn extra calories which in turn will help you to lose excess weight. A one hour workout will help you burn around 250-300 calories. So to lose one pound of fat, you need to burn 3500 calories - which means you need 14 days with hour-long workouts. Not exactly an encouraging statistic, huh? So you need to realize that exercise has many more benefits than as a simple weight loss tool. In fact, these other benefits are probably more important than the weight loss benefit.

Exercise keeps you healthy. Cardiovascular workouts will help build strength for your heart and lungs. Strength training workouts will build additional muscle mass (and we know we want to keep the muscle we have, right? See Rule 2). Weight bearing exercise will help strengthen bone, reducing the risk of osteoporosis (a risk factor after WLS). And regular activity will boost your HDL cholesterol levels - that's the "happy" cholesterol for which you want to see higher numbers. And let's not forget that exercise can reduce the risk of Type 2 Diabetes and some types of cancer.

Exercise is good for your mental well-being. When you exercise good chemicals are released - neurotransmitters and endorphins along with immune system boosting chemicals. These are the "feel good" chemicals that your body craves. Psychologists often prescribe exercise to depression patients and have seen positive results. Exercise can also serve as a release for pent-up emotions or aggression which can give a sense of mental peace. Exercise can also boost self-confidence, self-image and self-esteem. When you set your mind to a difficult task and work hard to achieve it, you gain the confidence because of that accomplishment.

Exercise boosts oxygen levels in your bloodstream, delivering added nutrients to body tissue. This simple action will give you more energy and pep in your step to accomplish the long list of tasks on your daily agenda.

What's Your Excuse?

Making excuses for not exercising is easy. Why is it so easy to blow off a workout? Even when I want to exercise I can still come up with an excuse to not do it. And often those excuses start out with: "I don't want to...." or "I don't feel like..." Right, nobody wants to exercise, nobody feels like getting all sweaty and running on a treadmill until you feel like you're going to puke up a lung.

And yes, I really do **want** to exercise. Well, more to the point... I want the results of what exercise will give me. A healthier body, weight loss, stronger muscles, a toned body, mental peace and self-confidence.

Excuses pile up little by little until one day you look around and realize you've been a slacker for far too long and it's time to get your butt back on track. What happens when you find yourself not working as hard as you should, not hitting the gym as often as you'd like, not sweating your butt off like you know you need to? Instead of five or six days of workouts, are you lucky to log two or three workouts a week. Have the excuses allowed you to be a slacker and now you don't know how to get back to a solid exercise routine?

How do I eliminate the excuses and do what I know I want and need to do for my own good health? Do like Nike and "Just Do It." Yeah, easier said than done, I know. There has to be a motivation behind just doing it. And my motivations for exercise must be bigger than the excuses.

Here are some motivations that will get you off the couch:

- I want to be healthier.
- I want to feel strong.
- I want to hit my goal weight.
- I want my body to be toned.
- I want to be able to do anything physical without hesitation or limitations.
- I want to be proud of myself.

Rule 6: Take your vitamins

Take vitamins every day for the rest of your life. This is a big rule and one with a lot of important reasons to back it up. I cover a lot of this information in other chapters, so I won't go into the all details of it again here.

We know that all along the digestive tract there are certain assigned points of absorption for various micronutrients (vitamins and minerals). Scientists are pretty smart and have figured out how the body breaks down, extracts and utilizes various vitamins and minerals and they've been able to pinpoint exactly how the body absorbs each of those nutrients. Those points of absorption will never grow back and the rest of the digestive tract will never be able to compensate fully for the bypassed sections that were eliminated during weight loss surgery.

In some cases there are certain micronutrients that have had all points of absorption eliminated completely. For instance, calcium has two main points of absorption in the small intestine. One in the duodenum and one is the upper jejunum - both of these spots have been eliminated in a typical RNY bypass of 100 centimeters. This means that any food we eat containing calcium, the nutrient will not be absorbed by the body. Therefore, we must get all our calcium needs from supplements that have already extracted the calcium from food sources and put it into a pill form that our body can immediately utilize.

The same is true for iron, Vitamin A, Vitamin E and others - all absorption points have been bypassed. Vitamin D has three main absorption points with two of them being bypassed. And some vitamins are no longer absorbed in the same way once certain factors are removed.

For instance, B12 requires the presence of Intrinsic Factor — a hormone produced in the lower part of the stomach (now bypassed). With Intrinsic Factor, B12 is extracted from the food we eat so that it can later be absorbed in the ileum (which is not bypassed). But if the extraction doesn't occur in the lower stomach, the absorption can't take place in the lower small intestine. Therefore, you have to take sublingual B12 (melts under the tongue) or get regular injections of B12 because you can no longer properly absorb B12 taken through oral supplements or from food.

Review the diagram in page 41 to understand more fully how this works and why vitamin supplements are so important after WLS.

Suffice it to say, you must take vitamin supplements for the rest of your life in order to remain healthy. You knew this was true before you hopped on the operating table. You signed up for it. No use whining and crying about it now — it's something you need to deal with forever.

Rule 7: No alcohol

Each surgeon has different rules about alcohol after bariatric surgery. Some say to wait six months or a year before trying any type of alcohol. Some say no alcohol, ever, for the rest of your life. What you must understand is that alcohol is metabolized differently now that you don't have a normal stomach. So you must first understand how alcohol affects you, and then decide which path you need to take on drinking after weight loss surgery.

How is alcohol digested in the non-WLS digestive system?

Unlike food, alcohol does not require any type of digestion before it is absorbed by the body. About 20 percent is absorbed directly across the walls of an empty stomach and can reach the brain within one minute. Once alcohol reaches the normal, non-WLS stomach, it begins to break down the alcohol immediately. This digestive process reduces the amount of alcohol entering the blood by approximately 20 percent. In addition, about 10 percent of the alcohol is expelled in the breath and urine.

So by this time a normal digestive system is only dealing with about 50 percent of the alcohol it first took in — 20 percent absorbed, 30 percent unused. The rest of the alcohol leaves the stomach and is quickly absorbed in the upper intestine straight into the bloodstream and forcing the liver to metabolize alcohol before anything else the liver is working on.

How is alcohol digested in a WLS digestive system?

Alcohol does not remain in the pouch after you drink it. Your pouch is a funnel shape and any fluid goes straight through without stopping. The alcohol isn't stored in the pouch long enough for any of it to be expelled in your breath and you don't get the benefit of lost alcohol through the digestive process. So the alcohol you drink is passed through to the small intestine where absorption happens immediately. This means that 100 percent of the alcohol you drink goes straight to the bloodstream and transported to the brain immediately. Essentially one alcoholic drink by a RNY patient is the same as two drinks by a normal digestive person.

Let's not forget the liver

Your liver has some pretty important functions in your body. Not only does it produce bile to aid in food digestion, but it also acts like the body's cleaning crew - filtering impurities from the blood and scrubbing the body of residual chemicals from medications. Many vitamins are stored in the liver, such as

Vitamins A, D and B12. The liver also makes cholesterol, processes fat for energy and turns glucose into glycogen. The liver is one of those important organs — one you can't live without and when it's damaged, life can get pretty yucky. So you want to do everything you can to protect your liver.

The liver has a lot of stuff on its To-Do List, right? But when you drink alcohol and that alcohol is coursing through your bloodstream, the liver must drop everything it is doing to deal with the chemicals you've introduced to the blood. Alcohol metabolism takes first priority for the liver. Alcohol metabolism permanently changes liver cell structure, which impairs the liver's ability to metabolize fats. So if you're damaging the liver in this way and you're trying to lose weight by asking the liver to process excess fat... what do you think is going to happen? Right. Fatty deposits in the liver. We already battle nonalcoholic fatty liver disease as morbidly obese people and we're doing everything in our power to repair the damage we've done to our bodies through obesity. So adding alcoholic-based fatty liver disease on top of the nonalcoholic fatty liver is not such a smart move, huh?

"But it's only one drink!" Unfortunately, that argument doesn't fly because science has shown that even one day of drinking can cause fatty deposits in the liver. And as you damage more and more liver cells, those fatty deposits will continue to get worse and worse.

Rule 8: No caffeine

Caffeine in coffee, tea and soda is another point of contention. Some doctors say no caffeine ever for the rest of your life - drink decaf instead. Some say we should limit it to one cup of coffee a day. Some clear you for caffeine, in moderation, after a set period of time - 6 or 12 months. Others have no rules whatsoever about the topic. No matter what your doctor says, it's important to understand the issues surrounding caffeine.

- for some, caffeine can be an appetite stimulant
- for some, caffeine can be an appetite suppressant
- for some, caffeine can cause stomach upset and digestive discomfort
- for some, caffeine can promote ulcers or thinning of the lining in the stomach
- for some, caffeine aids in gastric motility (keeps you regular)
- for some, caffeine can increase heart rates and blood pressure

- in large amounts (over 400mg/day or 32oz brewed coffee) caffeine can cause dehydration
- caffeine can interfere with calcium absorption if taken in large amounts (300mg/day or 20oz)
- tannins in coffee (more so in tea) interferes with Vitamin B12 and iron absorption
- tannins also have Anti-Thiamin Factors (ATF) that will "eat" thiamin (Vitamin B1) from the body

I waited almost a year after my surgery to reintroduce coffee to my diet. Before that I just drank decaf. I knew that coffee was highly acidic and I didn't want to damage my newly healing pouch — so I stayed away for as long as I could. When I started drinking coffee again, I took the above list of issues into consideration and paid close attention to how my body would react to the caffeine.

I also limit my caffeine intake to no more than 300mg per day - which comes out to about 20 ounces of coffee. This will prevent the leaching of calcium and also is well below the level where dehydration becomes a factor. I notice that caffeine, for me, is an appetite suppressant and I had to make a conscious effort to remember to eat after drinking my morning coffee.

Because the tannins in coffee can interfere iron and B12 absorption, I am sure to keep my coffee drinking well away from the dose of those two supplements. I drink coffee in the morning but take the supplements in the late afternoon or evening.

If you decide to drink coffee or caffeinated tea, be sure to consult your doctor's orders before you start. And ask his reasons for the rule, of course.

Rule 9: No Straws. No Gum. No Carbonation. No Soda. No Coconut. No Backwards Somersaults off the Diving Board.

Sometimes we're given rules and they seem pretty silly because we can't figure out why the rule exists. Usually a rule is based in some sort of real-life experience that a surgeon or nutritionist has seen in their practice. Then that one isolated experience becomes a new rule for all their other patients. And suddenly other surgeons are picking up on those rules and before you know it, the rule has spread to the masses and can take on the urban legend proportions.

In this section I'll cover several random rules that have some basis in fact or science... but they might be sitting on some pretty dubious foundations.

No Straws

This rule is one that I actually received from my nutritionist. The reason I was given made sense, but the reason I see others given doesn't make much sense to me. Here are the reasons I've heard for this particular rule:

- You'll suck in too much air and your pouch will expand too much and you will feel discomfort.

- You'll take too big of gulps and be able to drink too much water at one time.

The "too much air" argument is a bit silly to me. If I feel too much air building up in my belly I have the ability to burp. If you experiment with how straws make you feel and adjust your behavior accordingly, you should be fine to use straws like a normal person.

When I was given the no straws rule at the time of my surgery, the rule was a "No straws for the rest of your life" type of rule, thankfully. Instead we were told that until we fully understood what a "sip" was that it was a good idea to avoid drinking through a straw. Sipping is important in the early weeks after surgery because too much liquid in one gulp can cause pain and a "reappearance" of that offending gulp. The nutritionist who gave us this advice in my pre-op nutrition class said that once we were five or six weeks out from surgery that we could resume straw usage, if we wanted to. This explanation made sense to me and I appreciated the straightforward information.

No Gum

One day a newly post-op patient was walking down the street while chewing a huge wad of Double Bubble when suddenly she stumbled on a crack in the sidewalk and accidentally swallowed her gum. Because it was such a large amount of gum, it got stuck in her stoma and she had to have emergency surgery to get it removed. To help other newbies learn from her mistake, it is now advised that all WLS patients never chew gum — not ever again in their whole life.

Or maybe this rule is based on the myth that it takes seven years for chewing gum to pass through the human digestive system. This means that our tiny pouch will be filled up with chewing gum in no time flat and we won't have room for the nutrients needed for survival. (Check Snopes.com, that myth has been debunked.)

I chew gum. Not Double Bubble and not huge wads of it. And when I walk, I'm careful not to stumble. I also am conscious to not swallow my gum (which used to be a pre-op habit that I've had to break). And I also have a self-imposed rule that when I am no longer paying attention to the gum I'm chewing in my mouth, it's time to spit it out - which goes back to a technique I used to break myself of the habit of swallowing my gum.

No Soda. No Carbonation (unless you let it go flat first).

This rule comes with a lot of controversy and passionate arguments. Not necessarily from surgeons, but from patients. Many surgeons have a rule of no carbonation — soda, beer, sparkling water. But the reasons for the rule are a bit obscure. I'll review the reasons I've heard and give my opinion on them.

"Carbonation can stretch your pouch." This is the most common reason given and one I absolutely don't agree with. The claim is that when carbonated beverages are "trapped" inside your pouch, the gases will expand the pouch and cause it to expand unnaturally and cause permanent damage. This could be true if the pouch were a closed environment. But we know that the pouch has two openings, one at the top and one at the bottom. We also know that fluid flows straight through without stopping. So to claim that carbonation will stretch the pouch goes against what our anatomy lessons teach us.

"Soda is a gateway drug." Before surgery many of us lived on soda — diet soda or full-sugar soda — as a primary source of fluid. So yes, if you have issues with controlling your intake of diet soda after surgery, it could be a problem with leading to other bad habits. Those bad habits might be going back to sugary soda or associating the drinking of soda with other eating habits that do not promote healthy lifestyle. For instance, if you only drank soda when you stopped at the corner convenience store and you always picked up a couple candy bars and a hotdog to go with your super giant fountain soda... then yes, that could pose a problem for you. Just be aware that re-introducing soda to your post-op diet might be a trigger for other habits that you're trying to change.

"Carbonation is fine as long as you let it go flat first." Again, I think this suggestion goes back to the problem of carbonation stretching your pouch - which we know can't possibly be true. And who likes flat soda anyway? That'd be a really good reason to not even drink it in the first place. Yuck!

There are a couple other issue with soda that we need to address — issues that could cause serious problems.

Phosphoric Acid — this flavoring is contained in many dark cola beverages, some select light sodas and even some bottled teas and flavored waters. Check the label. Phosphoric Acid interferes with the absorption of calcium in the body.

Acidity — Carbonated soda is highly acidic and can cause damage to a compromised stomach lining. Obviously, right after surgery when your new pouch is healing, you should avoid highly acidic beverages.

No Coconut.

Honestly, this one just made me laugh. But it was a serious rule that a patient received. When I asked her if she knew why she wasn't allowed to eat coconut for the rest of her life — her response was, "My surgeon said it was too fibrous." I wonder if he realizes that we're not eating the actual coconut husk, but the tender meat inside?

Then I asked my own surgeon's office if they had ever heard of this rule. I was surprised to learn that they are now advising patients against coconut too. When I asked why, it turns out they had a patient once who at a large amount of shredded coconut, which then formed a fibrous ball in her pouch and it required surgery to repair the damage. So my advice on coconut: Use moderation when eating coconut — don't eat so much of it that you require surgery to get it through your pouch. (And look for the unsweet kind, too.)

Rule 10: Follow the rules

In the early weeks after surgery we are given a lot of rules that we must follow. Your surgeon gives you these rules so you can remain complication-free and heal properly. No matter which rules you're given or how silly they might seem - in the first several weeks after surgery, follow all the rules. All of them!

As a newbie, you don't yet have the privilege to decide which rules you'll follow or not. So if the doctor tells you to be on a full liquid diet for four weeks after your surgery, then do it. Even if someone else you know only had four days of full liquids before progressing to the next food stage. It doesn't matter. Follow your surgeon's guidelines to the letter.

Yes, I might be flippant in some of these descriptions in this section. I'm not being flippant to encourage you to neglect the rules - not at all. This part is serious. My goal is to help you understand the reasons behind the rules so you can more faithfully follow them. Your surgeon wants you to be healthy and successful, so follow his rules. Your life depends upon it.

Chapter 6
Nutritional Needs: Macronutrients

The topic of nutrition after bariatric surgery is something that could fill a whole series of books and still not be fully understood. This section is an attempt to cover the most important and most asked about areas of nutrition and give you some insight into my own personal experiences and practices. We'll cover a bit about food and how our body uses those nutrients to give us energy and keep our bodies functioning. We'll also talk about vitamins and supplements that we need after weight loss surgery and why they are so important. And of course since we're talking about nutrition, we have to talk about eating, right?

There are two main types of nutrients — macro and micro. Micro-nutrients are vitamins and minerals in food and supplements. Macro-nutrients are protein, carbohydrates and fats in the food we eat. Our body needs both type of nutrients and it is important for us to understand how the body uses these nutrients after weight loss surgery and why so much emphasis is placed on some nutrients more than others.

Protein

We talked about protein in the last chapter and why it is important to focus on eating protein first at each meal. But understanding more about what protein is and why it's important will help us realize just how essential this nutrient really is. I'll also review some basics on protein supplement types and how to choose high quality protein-based foods.

Protein is the building block of all cell formation with about 40% of the body's protein found in muscle, 25% in the body's organs and the rest in skin and blood. When the body needs to repair damaged cells (like surgical wounds or a paper cut) or maintain lean muscle mass during rapid weight loss, it needs protein to do those tasks. Protein is a complex nutrient made up of 22 different amino acids. Some amino acids the body creates on its own and the rest you must get from food sources. However, the amino acids that are created within the body are dependent upon the eight food-source amino acids to complete the cell formation process that protein is responsible for. These eight amino acids are called "essential" because without them the body is not able to function properly for the long term.

Going an extended period of time without the essential amino acids of protein you face malnutrition, the inability to heal, decreased mental capacity and even death — along with many other symptoms mostly seen in undeveloped countries that don't have ready access to proper nutrition. However, protein deficiency can occur in developed countries with individuals who are not eating adequate amounts of nutrition or have some form of malabsorption of nutrients — like WLS patients. When you take into account malabsorption because of the physical gastric bypass of Roux-en-Y it is even more important to focus on protein as an essential part of your diet.

Protein Digestion

Let's take a quick look at how protein is digested in a normal digestive system. When you eat protein-based foods like steak, chicken, or soy, the body must first break down that food before it can extract the nutrients it needs. Protein digestion relies heavily on mixing food with gastric acid in the stomach and the strong stomach muscle contractions (churning) to break food into small particles. Then the protein nutrients are absorbed all along the entire 20 to 25 feet of small intestine as food moves along the tract; however most absorption occurs in the proximal small intestine (which is the upper portion).

After a malabsorptive weight loss surgery, a much different digestive process takes place than what is described above.

After Roux-en-Y surgery you now have a small gastric pouch that produces very little (if any) gastric acid. The upper portion of your small intestine has also been bypassed and food no longer passes through this section.

Your small intestine is 20 to 25 feet long and the typical RNY bypass is 3 to 5 feet, so you still have about 15-20 feet of intestine for absorption. Although this is a significant amount of intestine for absorption, it's still 25% less than what you started with.

Gastric acid is still produced in the bypassed stomach and is sent down the bypassed small intestine and eventually the gastric acid meets up with the food you eat, but food is in your system for a while before the two mingle.

As you can see, protein digestion is significantly changed after WLS, which means you have to do some of the work that the stomach used to do for you. The primary work you need to do is chewing. Because the stomach no longer churns your food to break it down into small pieces, you have to be extra careful to chew your food well before swallowing. Remember in biology class we learned that digestion begins in the mouth? That is never truer now that we have to do a significant part of the stomach's job now.

How much protein do we need?

The ASMBS recommends RNY patients get about 70 grams of protein per day __or__ to calculate exact protein needs using a formula of 1.0 to 1.5 grams per kilogram of ideal body weight. Patients who had DS surgery need about 30% more than the RNY calculation due to increase malabsorption with their surgery type. What does that mean in laymen's terms? Let's use me as an example:

According to the BMI chart, my ideal body weight is 135 pounds (BMI of 21.7 - I stand 5'6" tall), so that would be 61 kilograms. Using the calculation of 1.0 to 1.5 grams per kilogram of ideal body weight, my daily protein requirement should be 61 grams to 92 grams.

Of course, our protein intake requirements are also dependent on our lab test results. For instance, I regularly see low-normal lab results for my protein, albumin and prealbumin tests; therefore, I must eat more protein than the standard recommendation so I don't become protein deficient. On average, I aim for around 100 grams of protein per day for my own optimal health.

In the early weeks and months after WLS you will be faced with the challenge of eating enough protein to meet your body's demand. Your tiny new stomach simply can't hold enough food to get all the protein you need. For instance, to get 70 grams of protein from food alone you would need to eat about 10 ounces of lean meat (there is approximately 7 grams protein per one-ounce of meat). Or drink almost nine cups of milk or eat three cups of cottage cheese. Obviously with a one-ounce sized pouch, these food volumes are impossible.

Protein supplements provide a significant amount of nutrition in a small amount of food volume. Therefore, it is often recommended that patients use some type of supplement in the early months after surgery. Some surgeons like their patients to stop using supplements after a set period of time whereas other surgeons recommend the use of protein supplements for life.

No matter which recommendation you receive from your medical team, discuss your individual eating plan, food intolerances and meal capacity with your doctor to ensure you're getting the protein your body requires. If you cannot eat enough food-based protein to meet your protein goals, continuing to use protein shakes to supplement your meals is a healthy and intelligent option.

I am over five years post-op and I still drink a protein supplement most days even though I'm able to eat enough food to reach my protein goal. I choose to use a supplement because it is convenient to my daily schedule and I simply enjoy the flavor of my morning Hot Protein Chai Tea (or whatever new recipe I've concocted). So I get about 75 grams of protein from the food I eat and about 25 grams of protein from a supplement.

Debunking the 30-gram Myth

There is a common myth that people can only absorb 30g of protein per meal. In fact, it's so widespread that I've even heard medical professionals quote this "fact" when giving advice to weight loss surgery patients. There is simply no evidence to support such a claim. In fact the ASMBS makes a point of addressing this myth in their bariatric nutrition literature to say: "One popular myth is that only 30 g/hr of protein can be absorbed. Although this is commonly found in both lay and some professional reports, there is no scientific basis for this claim. It is possible that, from a volume standpoint, patients might only realistically consume 30 g/meal of protein during the first year."

But, there's a but! Even though the body can easily absorb more than 30 grams in one meal, the body actually likes to receive nutrition at regular intervals. Which means, rather than consume 100 grams protein for breakfast and none the rest of the day, you want to evenly distribute your protein intake so your body had a steady supply of protein all day long. The best way to determine this is to use simple math. Calculate how much protein you need to consume for the whole day and then divide it by how many meals and snacks you have planned. If you aim for 80 grams of protein, then you'll budget 20 grams at breakfast, lunch and dinner, then 10 grams for a snack.

Types of Protein Supplements

Understanding the different types of protein supplements is essential in choosing the right one for you. Once you know the type of protein supplement you should use, then the hard work begins in finding a supplement you enjoy. There are literally thousands of different brands and flavors on the market today so finding the one you enjoy is a huge game of experimentation and requires lots of patience and creativity.

Whey Isolate Protein — this is the highest quality form of whey protein powder. Whey begins as cow's milk and then all the fat and lactose (sugar) is removed and you're left with just the protein. When you look at the label you'll see about 25g of protein per "scoop" (usually about 28g) with 0g carb and 0g fat. Because Whey Isolate is the highest quality, you're also going to pay more for it.

Whey Concentrate Protein — although still a high quality form of protein powder, it has not been processed as much as Isolate and you'll find that some fat and lactose still remain in the product. Not much, but still some. Typically you'll see Whey Concentrate containing about 1g-9g of fat and 1g-9g of carb (lactose) per serving. Check the labels carefully because some forms of Concentrate are higher quality than others. Because it's not as high a quality of blend, it's usually priced much cheaper. However, if you are lactose intolerant, you want to stick with Isolate instead.

Isolate vs. Concentrate — Whey Isolate Protein and Whey Concentrate Protein are exactly the same protein. The protein itself has the exact same quality, digestibility, bioavailability and Protein Digestibility Corrected Amino Acid (PDCAAS) score. The protein is the same. The only difference is that Whey Concentrate has a few extra "things" left in with the protein. So don't be fooled by those who say you can only use Whey Isolate Protein. That's a myth. You can use either form - they are exactly the same protein. However, if you have a lactose or fat intolerance, then stick with Isolate.

Protein Blends — A common way to achieve a high quality protein supplement while still maintaining an economical price point is to use a combination of both Whey Isolate and Concentrate. Check the label carefully to see which form of protein is listed first on the ingredient list. As with all nutrition and ingredients lists, the ingredients are listed by the order of quantity in the product. If Isolate is listed first, you'll likely see a lesser amount of fat and lactose on the nutrition label. I personally use a supplement that is a blend of whey Isolate and Concentrate.

Other Protein Types — some people find that they are actually "whey intolerant" and have to search for other types of protein supplements. There are definitely other options, but the variety is much more limited. Soy protein, rice protein, egg protein - all these powders can be purchased in the same way as whey protein although selection and availability is limited.

Protein Supplements to Avoid — stay away from the types of protein supplements that do not include all essential amino acids or are incomplete proteins. Specifically, collagen protein and hydrolyze protein sources. The ASMBS cautions that even collagen-based protein supplements that add other complete sources of protein to their supplements are still not considered complete proteins with the correct essential amino acids ratios. This type of supplement is found in a liquid or gelatin type product that promises significant protein content in a tiny amount of liquid such as the "protein shots" or "protein bullets" that give 40 grams of protein in 3 ounces of liquid. Avoid these products!

Experimenting with Protein Supplements

Because there are so many different brands and flavors of protein supplements it is often a difficult process to find a product that you enjoy using. Protein supplements can be expensive, so buying a large jar of protein powder every time you want to test a new flavor is not the ideal scenario. Thankfully there are several companies who sell samples of protein powders so you can try it before you buy a big jar of – refer to the Resources section at the back of the book for sources to buy protein powder samples online. I had to try about four dozen different brands/flavors in the first couple months after my surgery before I found two or three brands that worked for me.

There are two main types of protein supplements — powders and ready-to-drink (RTD) beverages. When choosing a RTD protein shake, pay careful attention to the ingredient list to ensure you're getting a quality protein supplement without significant added sugar or chemicals. Some popular options for RTD protein shakes include Muscle Milk Light; Isopure clear protein; Isopure Smoothie; Slim Fast Low-Carb; Premier Protein; Pure Protein; Oh Yeah!; EAS and many more.

Dry protein supplements – protein powder – need to be mixed into something else before you consume it. You can make it into a protein shake or mix it into whatever food you are eating for a meal to give it a boost of extra protein. There are dozens of different ways to mix protein powder and there are thousands of recipes available for experimenting. You can use unflavored protein or any of the dozens of flavors to compliment the recipe you're using. For instance, you might mix unflavored protein into your oatmeal but you want the distinct peach flavor when you mix a fun protein shake so you use Syntrax Nectar Fuzzy Navel Whey Isolate protein powder. The combinations are only limited by your imagination.

Protein Quality

A lot of emphasis is placed on protein supplements in the early months after surgery – likely because it is a new experience for most people so there are lots of questions about taste, texture, and recipes. But you can't discount the fact that getting your protein requirement from food is the ultimate goal after WLS. Food-based protein sources serve several different purposes. Of course, it provides you with the protein nutrients the body needs and the thermic effect of protein digestion is a huge benefit (the body burns calories as it digests food).

When you choose the type of protein supplement or food it is important to take into consideration the quality of that particular protein source.

The medical and scientific industry uses a standard method to measure protein quality called Protein Digestibility Corrected Amino Acid Score (PDCAAS) and each food is assigned a number based on how well the body is able to actually use the protein within the food. The scale ranges from 0 to 1.00 with 1 being a perfect score.

Creative ways to mix your protein powder

- Mix it with water
- Mix it with milk
- Mix it with soy milk
- Mix it with crystal light
- Mix it with diet juice
- Mix it with coffee
- Mix it with tea
- Mix it with hot cocoa
- Make it hot
- Make it cold
- Make it frozen
- Make it thin and serve it over ice
- Make it thick like a milkshake
- Make it thicker like pudding
- Mix it into yogurt
- Mix it into cottage cheese
- Mix in some fruit
- Mix in some spices
- Mix in some flavored sugar free coffee syrups
- Mix it into pudding
- Mix it into oatmeal
- Make it into protein bars
- Make it into dessert

Protein Quality Score of Select Foods

1.00	milk
1.00	egg
1.00	soy protein
1.00	whey protein
0.92	beef
0.91	soybeans
0.78	chickpeas
0.76	fruits
0.73	vegetables
0.70	legumes
0.59	cereals
0.42	whole wheat
0.25	wheat gluten protein

PDCAAS based on scale of 0 to 1.00 with 1.00 being a perfect protein.

Therefore it is important to remember that just because you see protein listed on a nutrition label doesn't mean you're getting 100% of the benefit of that protein. A bowl of bean soup that has 10g of protein, for instance, would have a PDCAAS score of .70 and would actually only give your body about 7g of useable protein.

There are many online calculators that will help you determine the PDCAAS of various types of foods as long as you have the full amino acid profile available for that food. Reputable protein powder manufacturers will publish their amino acid profiles on their websites or directly on their product labels. If a company is unwilling to provide this information, be wary of the products they are selling and proceed with caution.

Protein is an important nutrient for WLS patients. Understanding how the body uses it and why it is essential will help you remain healthy.

Carbohydrates

Carbohydrates (carbs) can be separated into two main categories: simple and complex. Some people call them bad carbs and good carbs but I personally prefer to not call any food "bad." There are no bad foods (or evil foods) - food is just food. We need to focus less on the moral standing of food and focus more on making the right choices that are healthiest for our bodies. So we'll stick with the terms simple carbs and complex carbs for now.

Simple Carbs are digested quickly. Many simple carbohydrates contain refined sugars and few essential vitamins and minerals. Some examples include: sweet treats (cake, cookies), high-sugar fruits (pineapple, bananas), "white stuff" (white bread, pasta, rice, potatoes, sugar) and most things that come in a box or are highly processed.

Complex Carbs take longer to digest. Most complex carbohydrates are packed with fiber, vitamins, and minerals. Examples are vegetables, low-sugar fruits (berries), whole grain starches, legumes and beans, and dairy — the more natural and whole the food, the more likely it is to be a complex carb.

After WLS you want to avoid the simple carb category except in extreme moderation. Just because you have WLS doesn't mean you're never allowed to have another Christmas cookie — but you can't make simple carbs a part of your everyday eating plan. Instead you should focus on complex carbs that are more wholesome and packed with fiber and nutrients.

The body needs carbs for proper function. The brain alone needs about 40 grams of carbs per day for clear thinking and rapid nerve response - and other vital organs in your body prefer to get their energy from glucose (which is the type of energy that carbohydrates become when they are digested). Studies have shown that anything less than 100 grams of carbs per day is considered a low-carb diet and can put your body into ketosis (which is not desirable for long periods of time).

Of course in the early weeks after surgery it is impossible to eat that many carbs and your sole focus should be protein and water and the amount of carbohydrates your surgeon's plan allows. But once you're several months out from surgery and able to eat a larger variety of foods, you can gradually increase carb intake to keep your body happy and functioning properly. Depending on your exercise level and overall calorie intake, you'll adjust your individual carb requirements with the help of your nutritionist or surgeon.

I shoot for about 35-40% of my calories to come from carbs. At 1400 calories a day that translates to 140 grams per day (there are 4 calories in each gram of carbohydrates) additionally I aim for 40% of my calories to come from protein and 20-25% from fat and try to get 25-30 grams fiber per day. My primary sources of carbs include vegetables, fruits, dairy, beans/legumes and whole grain starches.

Also remember that within the nutrition label there are several things listed under the carb category: Fiber, Sugar and Sugar Alcohol. Fiber is essential and the higher the number the better. Sugar we want to limit, of course, and I shoot for less than 10 grams per meal/snack. Sugar Alcohol, in theory, is not absorbed by the body so you don't need to worry about those, but many people have problems with sugar alcohol and it can cause gas, bloating or diarrhea, so be careful with this one.

The only way to really know what the true carbohydrates in a food include is to look at the ingredient list. Over time as you learn more and more about what different foods/ingredients are and their nutrient make up, you'll be able to recognize which things are carbs, proteins or fats. And when you spot a carbohydrate in the ingredient list, you'll eventually be able to automatically categorize it in your mind as simple or complex. It takes practice and there's a learning curve to it - but it's a valuable skill to have and worth the effort to learn.

Right after my surgery when I was so obsessed with food, I'd go on field trips to the grocery store. Leaving my wallet in the car I'd just go in and walk the aisles and read labels of different types of foods to understand them better. I'd do a bit of research at home on a certain nutrient, and then I'd go around the store looking at labels to see how that nutrient was used in various foods. One day I did a sodium field trip, one day a carb field trip, one day a whole grain tour - that's the best way to learn this stuff. Just soak in as much as you can. Nutrition is a learning process. Learn a little bit each day and before long you'll be comfortable with picking the right foods for your overall good health.

Sugar

Sugar is a carbohydrate and is listed on nutrition labels as an indented sub-section of carbs. When you look at the total amount of carbs on the label, the sugar grams are included in that total. But you need to look beyond the nutrition label to truly understand what kind of sugar is in the food. The ingredient list will reveal if it is the type of sugar we want to avoid, or if it is okay for us as WLS patients.

RNY patients are warned to stay away from sugar because of the risk of dumping syndrome. Other weight loss surgery patients are warned to avoid the extra calories in foods with excess sugar. But the problem with this advice is that all sugar is not created equally and understanding the different types of sugar can be a daunting task. There are more than 30 different names for sugar, according to Ann Louise Gittleman, author of "Get the Sugar Out," so we have to learn to understanding which sugars we should avoid and which are okay.

There are two main types of sugar – naturally occurring sugar and added sugar. Naturally occurring sugars are found in whole foods like fruit, milk and vegetables. The most common types of naturally occurring sugars are fructose (found in fruit) and lactose (found in milk). These types of sugars are generally not a problem for most WLS patients and will not cause dumping syndrome.

(We'll talk about lactose intolerance in a minute.) If you look at the nutrition label and see sugar grams listed, but don't see any form of sugar in the ingredient list, then it is probably a naturally occurring sugar.

"Added sugar" is the type of sweetener added to processed foods, beverages and sweet treats. This is the type of sugar we need to avoid. Look for names like corn syrup, cane crystals, dextrose, sucrose, maltodextrin, high fructose corn syrup, raw and turbinado sugar.

Lactose Intolerance

Since lactose falls into the carbohydrate category, I'll mention it briefly here.

Lactose intolerance is the inability to digest lactose – the sugar in milk products. Symptoms of lactose intolerance look a lot like dumping syndrome and it is often confused for dumping. You'll experience nausea, cramping and bloating, gas and diarrhea that usually beings within 30 minutes of eating or drinking lactose.

There are certain ethnic groups that are already at high risk for lactose intolerance. About 75% of African-Americans and Native Americans are lactose intolerance and about 90% of people of Asian descent. So that's strike one against me from the beginning – my Native American heritage should have made me lactose intolerance even before surgery, but I wasn't.

It is very common after RNY surgery for patients to suddenly become lactose intolerance. My sister had RNY ten years ago - she's lactose intolerant. My mom had RNY eights years ago - she's lactose intolerant. So when I had my RNY I fully expected to also be lactose intolerant. In fact, for the first four months after my surgery I was too scared to drink milk so I would only use soy milk. But somehow I got lucky because milk and I are friends.

Lactose intolerance happens after Roux-en-Y gastric bypass surgery because the portion of the small intestine that is bypassed is responsible for producing the digestive enzyme that processes milk – called lactase. Without that enzyme to break down the lactose into a simpler form that can be used by the body, the body will reject the lactose and will rush to get rid of it quickly. We know that the first part of the small intestine (first 3 to 5 feet) is bypassed and any enzymes produced in that portion won't mix with food until further down in the digestive tract. So by the time the milk and enzyme mix, the intolerance symptoms have already begun.

I suggest you use an alternative to milk in the early weeks after sugary. Soy, almond or rice milk are all good options. Then after you have established eating routines and are ready to experiment with milk, you can test the waters cautiously to find out your tolerance level.

Fats

When we eat excess calories, the body can make its own fat which is a type of storage system for future energy needs. We are all intimately aware of this kind of fat and the battle we all face to get rid of that body fat. But in this section I'm not going to talk about that kind of fat, I'll cover dietary fat — the type of macronutrient found in plants and animals and contained in the food that we eat.

Just like carbs, dietary fat has been called evil for so long that most chronic dieters are afraid of it. There is also a lot of misinformation floating around about fats and its time we start treating fats in our diet with the respect it deserves. Oh sure, there are some types of fats that we want to avoid but there are many types of fats that we need to eat in order maintain a healthy body.

There are healthy fats and unhealthy fats and of course, we want to choose healthy fats and avoid unhealthy fats as often as possible. It is impossible to avoid all unhealthy fat, but if we are aware of what types of foods contain which types of fat, we are better equipped to make good choices.

Unhealthy Fat

Saturated fats are found in animal-based foods such as beef, pork, butter and full-fat cheese or milk. These types of fat sources can contribute to increased LDL cholesterol levels which can lead to heart disease. Saturated fats should be consumed in moderation. Trans fats are also found naturally in animal sources of food, but more commonly they are man-made through a process of turning healthy fats into unhealthy fats through partial hydrogenation to make them more shelf-stable. This means when you look at a product label and see the term "partially hydrogenated vegetable oil," you need to put that product back on the shelf and choose something else.

Healthy Fat

There are many functions of the body that rely on adequate fat intake from your diet. Things like joint lubrication, good digestive health, vitamin absorption and organ function rely on getting enough healthy fats in your diet. Remember that fat-soluble vitamins (Vitamin A, D, E and K) rely on healthy sources of fat for proper break down, transport and absorption. Some good sources of healthy fat would include nuts and seeds, salmon or mackerel, some oils and avocado.

Polyunsaturated fats, which include Omega 3 fatty acids, help to lower bad cholesterol levels and promote good heart health. These types of fats are found in nuts and fish. Monounsaturated fats are primarily found in plant oils such as olive, sunflower seed, soy or canola oil. It is recommended that instead of sautéing foods in butter, to use olive oil instead.

Calories

The big difference between micronutrients and macronutrients is calories. Vitamins and minerals don't have calories. Protein, carbohydrate, and fat are where calories come from and we know that calories provide the body with the energy it needs to live, breath, move and function. Calories are a measure of energy. More specifically a calorie is a measurement of the amount of heat or energy needed to raise the temperature of one kilogram of water by one degree. So when you hear the phrase "burning calories" that is literally what's happening.

Each type of nutrient has a specific number of calories per gram and memorizing those number will help you better estimate how many calories are contained in the food you eat. Here's a quick cheat sheet:

Protein	4 calories per gram
Carbohydrates	4 calories per gram
Fat	7 calories per gram
Alcohol	9 calories per gram

An interesting tidbit about calories as it relates to weight loss surgery patients is what happens when we're not eating very many calories – like in the months following surgery. Have you experienced the cold feeling that so many of us do? No matter how many layers of clothes you put on, you're still shivering! I had my surgery in November and that first winter after my surgery was miserably cold for me. I wore layers and layers of clothes and invested in long johns to wear under my dress pants. That frigid feeling is related to two main things: 1) the loss of fat as we lose weight which acts as insulation for the body and 2) the intake of fewer calories which generates less body heat overall. This cold intolerance will stabilize over time as you get used to carrying around less weight and as you increase your calorie intake. The winter of my third year after surgery was much more bearable than that first year!

Chapter 7
Nutritional Needs: Micronutrients

Now that you know more than you ever thought you'd need to know about macronutrients — protein, carbohydrates and fats — it's time to learn about the micronutrients. Vitamins and minerals are called micronutrients because the body only needs micro amounts of these nutrients to sustain good health. Some of the larger mineral families are sometimes grouped into the macronutrient category, like calcium, but for the purposes of this writing we'll put all vitamins and minerals into the micronutrient groups.

I touched on vitamins a bit in previous chapters when we discussed the portion of the stomach and small intestine that is bypassed with Roux-en-Y so you understand how specific points within the small intestine have specifically assigned absorption tasks for vitamins and minerals contained in food. There are several key nutrients that are no longer normally absorbed which means WLS patients have an increased risk for deficiencies. Because the bypassed intestines will never again be able to absorb micronutrients normally, you need to continue your vitamin supplements for the rest of your life.

First, let's discuss the specific vitamin recommendations that the ASMBS lays out for bariatric patients. The vitamins listed below are where we start. Every patient should begin their WLS journey taking these vitamins and minerals but once you begin to get regular labs drawn you'll adjust your dose and vitamin routine based on what your body is demanding.

Which Vitamins When?

Some vitamins don't play well with other vitamins or minerals, so you have to carefully schedule your doses throughout the day to maximize the absorption of the supplements you take. Once you understand which vitamins need a

American Society of Metabolic and Bariatric Surgeons (ASMBS) Nutritional Guidelines

Suggested Postoperative Vitamin Supplements[13]

Consult your surgeon, primary care physician, or nutritionist for your personalized supplement plan.

	Adjustable Gastric Band	Roux-en-Y Gastric Bypass	Duodenal Switch
Multivitamin • Choose a high-potency vitamin containing 100% of daily value for at least 2/3 of nutrients • Begin with chewable or liquid and progress to whole tablet/capsule as tolerated • Avoid time-released supplements and avoid enteric coating • Choose a complete formula containing at least 18mg iron, 400mg folic acid, as well as selenium, and zinc in each serving • Avoid children's formulas which are incomplete	100% of daily RDA	200% of daily RDA	200% of daily RDA
Vitamin B12 • Sublingual tablets, liquid drops, mouth spray or nasal gel/spray	-	1000 ug/mo	-
• Intramuscular injection	-	350-500 ug/d	-
Elemental Calcium • Recommended dose amount is in addition to any food-based calcium sources • Calcium citrate and Vitamin D • Split into 500-600mg dose spaced evenly throughout day • Be mindful of serving size on supplement label • Do not combine calcium with iron containing supplements – wait 2 hours after taking multi-vitamin or iron supplement	1500 mg/d	1500-2000 mg/d	1800-2000 mg/d

Elemental Iron • Recommended for menstruating women and those at risk for anemia • Avoid enteric coating • Do not mix iron and calcium supplements, take 2 hours apart • Avoid excess intake of tea due to tannin interaction • Encourage foods rich in heme iron • Vitamin C may enhance absorption of non-heme iron sources	-	18-27 mg/d elemental	18-27 mg/day elemental
Fat Soluble Vitamins • Water-soluble preparations of fat-soluble vitamins are available and best absorbed • Retinol sources of Vitamin A should be used to calculate dosage • With all procedures, higher maintenance doses may be required for those with a history of deficiency	- - -	- - -	Vit A – 10,000IU Vit D – 2,000IU Vit K – 300 ug
B-Complex • B-50 dosage • Avoid time release. Liquid form available. • No known risk of toxicity	I per day	I per day	I per day

cushion of time surrounding its dose, you can begin to build your own vitamin schedule. These are the basic interaction rules when figuring out when to take your vitamins:

• **Calcium and Vitamin D are Friends** — take them together, they help each other absorb better.

• **Iron and Vitamin C are Friends** — Iron needs an acid environment to break down and Vitamin C does that job so make sure they are in your tummy at the same time. Iron does not like food, so take it on an empty stomach. However, if you get an upset tummy because of the iron, pick a small non-dairy snack.

- **Iron and Calcium are Enemies** — iron and calcium fight for the same cell receptors in the body and calcium is bigger and "meaner" so always wins. Which means the iron is simply excreted from the body and not used at all. Keep iron and calcium at least 2 hours apart from each other.

- **Calcium in Small Doses** — Your body can only deal with 500-600mg of calcium at a time, so split up your doses into three or four time per day to reach your 1500-2000mg daily goal. Calcium tends to absorb better when taken with a meal, so schedule it that way if you can.

- **Vitamin B's are a Family** — they work together as a team and are best taken at the same time. Your multi-vitamin has many B's in it, so take it together with your Vitamin B12, B-complex and any other specialize B Vitamins you're taking.

So in summary, we have to keep iron and calcium at least two hours apart from each other. Iron likes to be taken on an empty acidic stomach and calcium likes to be taken with food. We have to keep calcium doses to no more than 500-600mg per dose and spread at least two hours apart from each other. It is also recommended that we split up the two daily multivitamin doses so they aren't taken at the same time. And if you happen to be taking a medication that also has a set of rules of its own, there are even more dosing times to work around. That's a lot of rules to remember! Consult your nutritionist, she can help with your schedule.

Micronutrient: The Details

There is some specific information about some vitamins and minerals that I feel is important for all WLS patients to know and understand. It is not enough to simply know that you must take vitamins for the rest of your life, you should also understand why. Just like I said in The Rules have a Reason in Chapter 5, sometimes it helps us follow the rules more faithfully if we truly understand why the rules are so important.

For instance, do you know why it is important we use calcium citrate instead of calcium carbonate? Or why we should use sublingual Vitamin B12 instead of an oral supplement? Do you understand how Vitamin D, Calcium and your parathyroid all work together to maintain proper bone density? Do you understand what all the different types of iron are and which one is best for you? These are a few of the questions that I'll answer in this section.

The information I cover in this section is an attempt to give you a high-level overview, in layman's terms, of the complex information about micronutrients. If you have specific questions about your own lab results, vitamin schedules, or nutritional needs definitely consult your surgeon, primary care physician, or bariatric nutritionist.

Calcium Citrate

It's very important that after WLS that we take calcium citrate, not calcium carbonate. Carbonate is the most readily available type of supplement on store shelves, but it is not the right kind of calcium for WLS patients.

Calcium Citrate is the most soluble in a non-acid environment. After surgery there is no longer a significant amount of gastric acid in your stomach pouch and what little that is there is often suppressed with acid blockers prescribed by your surgeon. The cheaper and more readily available form of calcium - which is carbonate - requires gastric acid to be broken down within the stomach and absorbed by the intestines.

There's a medical condition called Achlorhydria — which is when a patient no longer produces stomach acid (hydrochloric acid). By studying this condition we can learn a lot about how we, as post-RNY patients, should be treated by our doctors and which medications and supplements we need to choose.

In a study published in the New England Journal of Medicine by R.R. Rekker[14] the calcium absorption rate of achlorhydria patients was studied. After giving test subjects a dose of calcium, the bioavailability (absorption of the dose) was measured. It's clear that after gastric bypass surgery we must take calcium citrate to have a chance at keeping healthy bones and teeth. His findings were:

Calcium Carbonate Absorption = 4%
Calcium Citrate Absorption = 45%

As we saw in the chart of vitamin requirements earlier in this chapter, RNY patients need 1500-2000mg of calcium citrate per day, in addition to any calcium we get from food. We also know that the body can only use 500-600mg calcium in a two-hour timeframe. So that means you have to schedule three or four doses of calcium throughout the day to get all your calcium in.

Protecting Your Bones

Osteoporosis is a known complication of gastric bypass surgery because of the body's decreased ability to absorb calcium. Only about 1% of the body's calcium is found in the blood, the other 99% is found in bones, teeth and tissue.

So when you have labs drawn to check for calcium levels, it is only testing 1% of your total calcium stores. The 1% of calcium in the blood is essential to sustaining life — it keeps the heart pumping and helps with nerve reflexes — so the body will do everything in its power to maintain a perfect blood calcium level. If you do not get enough calcium in your diet or through supplements, then the body will pull calcium from its storage (bones, teeth, tissue) to keep the blood calcium levels within perfect range.

When you and your doctor look at your lab results, you can't judge if we're taking enough calcium by the number you see. Instead you have to look at a combination of factors that give you a clearer picture of how calcium is being used in the body. The most reliable method to determine if your body is using its calcium storage is having a DEXA Bone Density Scan to measure how strong your bones are. Based on the recommendation of the ASMBS, all weight loss surgery patients with malabsorptive surgeries should have a DEXA scan annually to monitor the health of your bones. The other way to see if your body is using the calcium you take is by looking at other lab results in combination with your calcium lab levels — Vitamin D and PTH, specifically.

Vitamin D aids in the absorption of calcium. A low Vitamin D lab level will not allow all the calcium you take to be properly absorbed. The parathyroid (PTH) gland (not related to the thyroid, just located next to it) is the gatekeeper of calcium. If the blood calcium levels drop too low, the PTH signals to the bones to release some stored calcium to the blood for immediate use. When you see a PTH lab result that shows a high level of PTH and a low level of Vitamin D — you can assume that the body is leaching calcium from your bones. If this cycle is allowed to continue for too long, you will develop osteoporosis.

Vitamin D

Vitamin D is often called the Sunshine Vitamin because the body can make Vitamin D through exposure to the sun. When your skin is exposed to ultraviolet light the cholesterol in your skin converts the sunlight to Vitamin D3 and is ready to be used by the body. However, depending on what time of year it is in your part of the world, you may not receive enough sun exposure to provide the right amount of Vitamin D.

Those of us who live in the Midwest (I'm in Michigan) are more likely to have Vitamin D deficiency than someone who lives in the tropics. Unfortunately, Vitamin D production from sun exposure is also hindered by excess body fat so we morbidly obese folks are at a greater disadvantage for proper Vitamin D synthesis. Studies show that pre-op WLS patients have Vitamin D deficiency in up to 80% of cases.[15]

If you have dark skin — African American, Asian, Latino, and Native American — you are also at an increased risk for Vitamin D deficiency because your skin pigment acts as a natural sunscreen and blocks the production of Vitamin D. In fact, one study showed that 95% of all African American pre-op WLS patients are Vitamin D deficient.[16]

Vitamin D is a fat soluble vitamin and there are two main types we need to worry about — ergocalciferol (Vitamin D2) and cholecalciferol (Vitamin D3). Vitamin D3 is made by the sun and found in some natural sources (like fish, eggs and meat). Vitamin D2 is the most common form of supplement you get from pills or added Vitamin D in foods (like milk).

Vitamin D3 is the active form of the vitamin and all Vitamin D2 supplements must be converted to D3 before it can be used. It is shown that during the conversion process from Vitamin D2 to Vitamin D3, the body wastes a portion of the D2 so it is automatically less potent when it's time for the body to actually use the Vitamin D. Vitamin D3 is approximately 87% more potent than Vitamin D2 in raising and maintaining serum D levels.[17] So, we obviously want to choose the better supplement to begin with.

Also note that in the ASMBS guidelines we are advised to choose a water soluble form of fat soluble vitamins. Typically when you buy a bottle of Vitamin D3 at the store it is little gel-caps filled with an oily substance. But after gastric bypass surgeries you will automatically malabsorb a certain amount of the fat you eat, so you want to avoid this type of supplement. Instead look for a water-miscible, or "dry," formula — which simply means that it is a pill made of compressed powder or a capsule filled with a powdery substance that will easily dissolve in water without the addition of any fat-based substance. There are several brands of supplements that offer the water soluble form of Vitamin D including Nature Made and BioTech. You will most likely need to buy these types of supplements online rather than finding them in a local store.

The current government recommendation for Vitamin D intake is very low (600 iu per day)[18] and has not been updated to match the newly emerging science that shows we need more. In fact, current statistics show that healthy adults with normal Vitamin D levels need about 5,000iu per day to maintain their good lab results.[19] Of course, we are not normal — or at least not normal-

gutted. We've been bypassed and we don't eat as much food containing Vitamin D as the normal population. So we need to take more Vitamin D than a normal healthy adult.

Many primary doctors have not learned about the latest research about Vitamin D and may still be recommending lower doses. It is our responsibility to make sure our medical staff is educated on how best to treat us as bariatric patients. Review the latest information at the Vitamin D Council's website and share that information with your doctors.

Another common problem we face is that when we are diagnosed as being Vitamin D deficient and doctors prescribed a mega-dose of Vitamin D, we are getting the wrong kind of Vitamin D. The only mega-dose prescription Vitamin D (50,000iu) available through your pharmacy is Vitamin D2 suspected in an oil-based gel-cap (usually a little green pill filled with an oily substance). Instead we need to purchase an over-the-counter Vitamin D3 water soluble formula that is better absorbed in a bypassed gut and is more potent than D2. Biotech is one of the few manufacturers who produce this mega-dose of dry Vitamin D3 and it is available for sale directly from their website or on Amazon.com. This is the brand I use and my doctor approves.

In the mid-1990's it was determined that labs begin using a standard measure of Vitamin D tests. However, results can be displayed in one of two different measurements – nanomoles per liter (nmol/L) and nanograms per milliliter (ng/mL). Emerging science is showing that Vitamin D lab results above 50nmol/L or above 20 ng/mL are helping patients realize many amazing health benefits such as reduced risk of certain cancers, inflammation leading to chronic diseases and a reduced risk of developing neuromuscular diseases such as muscular dystrophy. The National Institutes of Health provides the following guideline for evaluating Vitamin D lab results[20]

Vitamin D Lab Results Guidelines

nmol/L	ng/mL	Health status
<30	<12	Associated with vitamin D deficiency, leading to rickets in infants and children and osteomalacia in adults
30–50	12–20	Generally considered inadequate for bone and overall health in healthy individuals
≥50	≥20	Generally considered adequate for bone and overall health in healthy individuals

Source: National Institutes of Health

The previous chart is similar to what you'll see on your lab results report. But to better understand what this means, here is the information in layman's terms:

Vitamin D labs under 30nmol/L — you are at risk for osteomalacia (rickets) and osteoporosis because your body is not able to use the calcium you are giving it. Instead your body is excreting supplement calcium you take and pulling calcium from your bones instead. Calcium is essential to keep your heart beating, so your body will sacrifice your bones to keep you alive. With Vitamin D levels this low, your body is in crisis mode.

Vitamin D labs of 30-50nmol/L — your body is simply using it up as fast as you're putting it in. You're not getting any of the health benefits of Vitamin D with levels in this range.

Vitamin D labs over 50nmol/L — this is finally when your body begins to store some Vitamin D in your kidneys for other uses in the body. This should be your first milestone goal for lab levels.

Vitamin D labs 80-100nmol/L — finally you're getting the amazing benefits of Vitamin D. This is the range we want to stay in forever. With levels over 80 we see a 50% reduction in certain cancers (breast, cervical, prostate) and a reduction in the risk for Multiple Sclerosis and heart disease.

Vitamin B12

Vitamin B12 is a very important vitamin. In fact, it's so important that when you become deficient in Vitamin B12, it gets the medical term pernicious anemia – pernicious literally translates to "deadly" or "fatal." This important nutrient helps to regulate the nervous system, the beating of your heart, the creation of DNA in your body and even plays an essential role in metabolism of cells.

Vitamin B12 is found naturally in fish, meat and eggs so the general population doesn't have a problem getting enough B12 in their normal diets. However, after WLS it is estimated that Vitamin B12 deficiency affects as many as 25% of all Roux-en-Y patients. Why is deficiency high in RNY patients, but not in other surgery types? I'm glad you asked!

Review the diagram on page 41 and you'll see that Vitamin B12 has an assigned absorption point in the lower part of the small intestine which is still intact after Roux-en-Y. However, that absorption point relies on Vitamin B12 being properly prepared for absorption and without that preparation, the absorption can't happen. Vitamin B12 preparation happens because of Intrinsic Factor which is produced in the portion of the stomach that is bypassed in RNY patients. Intrinsic Factor is responsible for grabbing hold of B12 in the duodenum (upper small intestine that is bypassed) and transporting the Vitamin B12 to the ileum (lower small intestine) for absorption. Without Intrinsic Factor any Vitamin B12 we ingest is gobbled up by bacteria all along the intestinal walls, and that bacterium is hungry for this valuable nutrient.

There is believed to be some level of passive absorption that can happen without Intrinsic Factor — but the amount is only 1-3% and is different with different bodies. Therefore, we must use forms of Vitamin B12 that can be absorbed without the requirement of having Intrinsic Factor present. There are several options but the most common include sublingual pills that dissolve underneath the tongue or monthly intramuscular injections. Other options include nasal sprays and patches.

Some symptoms of Vitamin B12 deficiency — pernicious anemia — include fatigue, lack of energy, inability to concentrate, confusion and dementia, tingling or loss of feeling in hands and feet. The tingling or numbness in hands and feet that happens with pernicious anemia may become a permanent disability that cannot be reversed even after Vitamin B12 levels return to normal. I know of three friends in the WLS community who suffered permanent nerve damage because of Vitamin B12 deficiency; one will be confined to a wheel chair for the rest of her life.

Iron

Iron is a mineral that's found everywhere — the moon, meteorites, rocks, dirt, air, water, plants, and animals. Iron is an "essential" micronutrient that the body can't produce on its own and requires you to consume iron-rich foods to give you what it needs (that's why scientists use the term essential). Since we can't stop at the corner store and pick up an extra meteorite to gnaw on, we need to rely on plant and animal sources to get the iron we need. However, the assigned absorption points for iron are bypassed after RNY, so we must rely on iron from supplements to meet the daily needs.

Unlike other vitamins and minerals that work best when taken with food, iron likes an empty stomach for best absorption and doesn't like to be near any other vitamins. However, iron prefers an acidic environment, so you will probably be advised to take Vitamin C with iron.

Most of the iron in your body is responsible for carrying oxygen to all the tissues in your body. Some of the iron is tasked with supplying oxygen to muscle and some is stored for future use. Oxygen transport is job number one for iron and without adequate iron, tissue suffocates.

Iron is a very complex mineral and there are lots of pieces of the iron puzzle that all fit together seamlessly to give us a clear picture of what's happening inside the body. First, let's understand what types of iron are available over-the-counter and which one to choose for your supplement.

Iron Supplement Types

Iron Type	Brand Options	Information
Ferrous sulfate	• Feosol (ferrous sulfate) • Feratab • Fer-Iron • Slow Fe	Usually the cheapest form. Well absorbed. Can cause stomach cramping, nausea, vomiting, dark stools and constipation; less often diarrhea and heartburn.
Ferrous gluconate	• Fergon • Ferralet • Simron	Slightly more expensive from ferrous sulfate. Slightly fewer side effects.
Ferrous fumerate	• Femiron • Feostat • Ferro-Sequels • Fumasorb • Fumerin • Hemocyte	Similar to ferrous gluconate.
Polysacchairde iron	• Ferimin • Hytinic • Niferex • Nu-Iron • Poly Iron	May cause less nausea and constipation than other. Take with Vitamin C to increase absorption
Carbonyl Iron	• Feosol (carbonyl iron) • Sundown • Perfect Iron • Bifera	Least upsetting to digestive system. Does not cause nausea or constipation. Less toxic than ferrous forms of iron so patients can take 10-150 times the dose without side effects. Take with Vitamin C to increase absorption.
Proferrin	Proferrin	Designed to increase Ferritin levels only. (See the experiment done by Andrea at www.wlsvitagarten.com)

Source: Iron Disorders Institute

When you have labs drawn to check your iron levels, there are several different tests that make up the iron panel. The scientific explanation of each of these lab tests can be confusing, but there is an easy way to understand what they mean — just think of it all in terms of money.

Hemacrit and hemaglobin are like cash in your wallet. It's your readily expendable iron. Hemaglobin (hgb) is a protein that transports oxygen to the body. Hematocrit (hct) measures the proportion of blood volume that is occupied by red blood cells.

Iron saturation is like your savings account at your hometown bank that is stored for easy access in case you run low on cash.

Transferrin is like the armored truck that delivers new cash to the bank from the Federal Reserve. Transferrin is a protein that is the major transporter of iron and ideally is saturated with 25-35% iron; when working properly, transferrin binds to iron and transports it to all tissues, vital organs, and bone marrow so that normal metabolism, DNA synthesis, and red blood cell production can take place.

Total Iron Binding Capacity (TIBC) is the size of your armored truck. It is a measure of the maximum iron concentration that transferrin can bind. If you need a bigger armored truck, that means more money is being transferred at one time. Increased TIBC levels may indicate iron-deficiency anemia; decreased TIBC may indicate cirrhosis.

Ferritin is your 401k of iron. It's your long term iron storage. Ferritin is a protein that acts like a large holding vessel; contains iron that we don't presently need but if the hemacrit and hemoglobin run low and there's not enough iron saturation to replenish them — the body turns to ferritin for its iron needs. If you see your ferritin slowly being depleted over time and your transferrin oversaturated to keep the hemacrit and hemoglobin levels in range, you're facing some serious retirement problems that need to be dealt with aggressively. Never let your ferritin levels drop too close to the bottom of the range.

Vitamins and Labs for Life

There are other micronutrients that are important to WLS patients. However, what I've covered here represent the most common and essential supplements we'll need to take forever. Your vitamin regimen will depend entirely on your own personal lab results. That's why it is so important to stay on top of your labs for the rest of your life. Your surgeon's office will provide you a list of labs that need to be drawn and your primary care physician needs to be kept in the tight circle of your health care too. In fact, my surgeon's office requires that my labs be ordered by my primary doctor and that copies are sent to be included in my surgical file as a secondary measure.

When I get my labs drawn, (usually about 12-14 vials of blood!) I am always sure to get a hard copy of the results for my own personal files. I keep track of my individual test results on a master spreadsheet where I can see all my results side-by-side. This allows me to spot any downward trends in specific lab tests over time and then work with my doctors to get that trend corrected before it becomes a deficiency. Because of this proactive approach I have been fortunate to not have any major vitamin deficiencies since my surgery.

Another important tool I use is a chart that shows possible symptoms of common nutrient deficiencies. For instance if I notice my fingernails are suddenly starting to get weak, peel and brittle, I can quickly check this chart and see that it might be caused by low levels of calcium, iron or zinc. So this gives me some things to chat with my doctor about and to watch closely on my lab results. No, I wouldn't automatically increase my calcium, iron and zinc supplements (that would be dangerous), but it would give me a starting point for a conversation with my doctor.

The chart on the following pages should not be used as a diagnosis tool. Also, remember that foods rich in certain vitamins may not be fully absorbed by those who had a malabsorptive bariatric surgery. Refer to the diagram on page 41 to understand where certain micronutrients are absorbed and cross reference with the chart on page 80 for postoperative supplements recommended by the ASMBS.

Common Nutrient Deficiencies[21]

This information refers to the general population, not just the bariatric community. Also remember that after gastric bypass surgery we are not fully able to absorb micronutrients (vitamins and minerals) from the food we eat (see page 41) — thus the need to for a lifetime of taking vitamins and supplements. Do not use this information for self-diagnosis. Consult your health care professional for treatment. Use this information as a conversation starter with your physician.

Nutrient	Incidence of Deficiency	Typical Symptoms & Diseases	Natural Sources of Nutrient
Biotin	Uncommon	Dermatitis, eye inflammation, hair loss, loss of muscle control, insomnia, muscle weakness	chard, tomatoes, romaine lettuce, carrots, almonds, chicken eggs, onions, cabbage, cucumber, cauliflower, goat's milk, cow's milk, raspberries, strawberries, halibut, oats, and walnuts
Calcium	Average diet contains 40 to 50% of RDA	Brittle nails, cramps, delusions, depression, insomnia, irritability, osteoporosis, palpitations, periodontal disease, rickets, tooth decay	blackstrap molasses, Swiss chard, yogurt, kale, mozzarella cheese, cow's milk, goat's milk, basil, thyme, dill seed, cinnamon, and peppermint leaves, romaine lettuce, celery, broccoli, sesame seeds, fennel, cabbage, summer squash, green beans, garlic, tofu, Brussel sprouts, oranges, asparagus and crimini mushrooms
Chromium	90% of diets deficient	Anxiety, fatigue, glucose intolerance, adult-onset diabetes	romaine lettuce, onions, tomatoes, brewer's yeast, oysters, liver, whole grains, bran cereals, and potatoes
Copper	75% of diets deficient; average diet contains 50% of RDA	Anemia, arterial damage, depression, diarrhea, fatigue, fragile bones, hair loss, hyperthyroidism, weakness	calf's liver, crimini mushrooms, turnip greens, molasses, chard, spinach, sesame seeds, mustard greens, kale, summer squash, asparagus, eggplant, and cashews, peppermint, tomatoes, sunflower seeds, ginger, green beans, potato, tempeh
Omega 3 fatty acids	Very common	Diarrhea, dry skin and hair, hair loss, immune impairment, infertility, poor wound healing, premenstrual syndrome, acne, eczema, gall stones, liver degeneration	salmon, flax seeds and walnuts, scallops, cauliflower, cabbage, cloves and mustard seeds, halibut, shrimp, cod, tuna, soybeans, tofu, kale, collard greens, and brussels sprouts

Nutrient	Incidence of Deficiency	Typical Symptoms & Diseases	Natural Sources of Nutrient
Folic acid	Average diet contains 60% of RDA,; deficient in 100% of elderly in one study; deficient in 48% of adolescent girls; requirement doubles in pregnancy	Anemia, apathy, diarrhea, fatigue, headaches, insomnia, loss of appetite, neural tube defects in fetus, paranoia, shortness of breath, weakness	romaine lettuce, spinach, asparagus, turnip greens, mustard greens, calf's liver, parsley, collard greens, broccoli, cauliflower, beets, lentils, quash, black beans, pinto beans, garbanzo beans, papaya, string beans
Iodine	Uncommon since the introduction of salt with iodine	Cretinism, fatigue, hypothyroidism, weight gain	sea vegetables, yogurt, cow's milk, eggs, strawberries, mozzarella cheese
Iron	Most common mineral deficiency	Anemia, brittle nails, confusion, constipation, depression, dizziness, fatigue, headaches, inflamed tongue, mouth lesions	chard, spinach, thyme, turmeric, romaine lettuce, blackstrap molasses, tofu, mustard greens, turnip greens, string beans, shiitake mushrooms, beef tenderloin, lentils, brussel sprouts, asparagus, venison, garbanzo beans, broccoli, leeks, kelp
Magnesium	75 to 85% of diets deficient: average diet contains 50 to 60% of RDA	Anxiety, confusion, heart attack, hyperactivity, insomnia, nervousness, muscular irritability, restlessness, weakness	Swiss chard, spinach, mustard greens, summer squash, broccoli, blackstrap molasses, halibut, turnip greens, pumpkin seeds, peppermint, cucumber, green beans, celery, kale and a variety of seeds, including sunflower seeds, sesame seeds, flax seeds
Manganese	Unknown, may be common in women	Atherosclerosis, dizziness, elevated cholesterol, glucose intolerance, hearing loss, loss of muscle control, ringing in ears	mustard greens, kale, chard, raspberries, pineapple, romaine lettuce, spinach, collard greens, turnip greens, kale, maple syrup, molasses, garlic, grapes, summer squash, strawberries, oats, spelt, green beans, brown rice, garbanzo beans, ground cloves, cinnamon, thyme, peppermint, turmeric, leeks, tofu, broccoli, beets, whole wheat, tempeh, cucumber, peanuts, millet, barley, figs, bananas, kiwifruit, carrots, black beans

Nutrient	Incidence of Deficiency	Typical Symptoms & Diseases	Natural Sources of Nutrient
Pantothenic acid (Vitamin B5)	Average elderly diet contains 60% of RDA	Abdominal pains, burning feet, depression, eczema, fatigue, hair loss, immune impairment, insomnia, irritability, low blood pressure, muscle spasms, nausea, poor coordination	mushrooms, cauliflower, broccoli, calf's liver, turnip greens, sunflower seeds, tomato, strawberries, yogurt, eggs, winter squash, collard greens, chard and corn
Potassium	Commonly deficient in elderly	Acne, constipation, depression, edema, excessive water consumption, fatigue, glucose intolerance, high cholesterol levels, insomnia, mental impairment, muscle weakness, nervousness, poor reflexes	chard, crimini mushrooms, spinach, fennel, kale, mustard greens, brussel sprouts, broccoli, winter squash, blackstrap molasses, eggplant, cantaloupe, tomatoes, parsley, cucumber, bell pepper, turmeric, apricots, ginger root, strawberries, avocado, banana, tuna, halibut, cauliflower cabbage
Pyridoxine (Vitamin B6)	71% of male and 90% of female diets deficient	Acne, anemia, arthritis, eye inflammation, depression, dizziness, facial oiliness, fatigue, impaired wound healing, irritability, loss of appetite, loss of hair, mouth lesions, nausea	spinach, bell peppers, turnip greens, garlic, tuna, cauliflower, mustard greens, banana, celery, cabbage, crimini mushrooms, asparagus, broccoli, kale, collard greens, Brussels sprouts, cod, chard
Riboflavin (Vitamin B2)	Deficient in 30% of elderly Britons	Blurred vision, cataracts, depression, dermatitis, dizziness, hair loss, inflamed eyes, mouth lesions, nervousness, neurological symptoms (numbness, loss of sensation, "electric shock" sensations), seizures, sensitivity to light, sleepiness, weakness	mushrooms, calf liver, spinach, romaine lettuce, asparagus, chard, mustard greens, broccoli, collard greens venison, turnip greens, chicken eggs, yogurt, cow's milk
Selenium	Average diet contains 50% of RDA	Growth impairment, high cholesterol levels, increased incidence of cancer, pancreatic insufficiency (inability to secrete adequate amounts of digestive enzymes), immune impairment, liver impairment, male sterility	brazil nuts, button mushrooms, shiitake mushrooms, cod, shrimp, snapper, tuna, halibut, calf's liver, salmon, chicken's eggs, lamb, barley, sunflower seeds, turkey, mustard seeds, oats
Thiamin (Vitamin B1)	Commonly deficient in elderly	Confusion, constipation, digestive problems, irritability, loss of appetite, memory loss, nervousness, numbness of hands and feet, pain sensitivity, poor coordination, weakness	asparagus, romaine lettuce, mushrooms, spinach, sunflower seeds, tuna, green peas, tomatoes, eggplant and brussels sprouts.

Nutrient	Incidence of Deficiency	Typical Symptoms & Diseases	Natural Sources of Nutrient
Vitamin B12	Serum levels low in 25% of hospital patients	Anemia, constipation, depression, dizziness, fatigue, intestinal disturbances, headaches, irritability, loss of vibration sensation, low stomach acid, mental disturbances, moodiness, mouth lesions, numbness, spinal cord degeneration	Animal sources: snapper, calf's liver, venison, shrimp, scallops, salmon, and beef Plant sources are less consistently good sources of B-12: kelp, blue-green algae, brewer's yeast, tempeh, miso, tofu
Vitamin C	20 to 50% of diets deficient	Bleeding gums, depression, easy bruising, impaired wound healing, irritability, joint pains, loose teeth, malaise, tiredness.	broccoli, bell peppers, kale, cauliflower, strawberries, lemons, mustard and turnip greens, brussels sprouts, papaya, chard, cabbage, spinach, kiwifruit, snow peas, cantaloupe, oranges, grapefruit, limes, tomatoes, zucchini, raspberries, asparagus, celery, pineapples, lettuce, watermelon, fennel, peppermint and parsley
Vitamin D	62% of elderly women's diets deficient	Burning sensation in mouth, diarrhea, insomnia, myopia, nervousness, osteomalacia, osteoporosis, rickets, scalp sweating	natural sunlight, salmon, shrimp, Vitamin D fortified milk, cod, eggs
Vitamin E	23% of male and 15% of female diets deficient	Gait disturbances, poor reflexes, loss of position sense, loss of vibration sense, shortened red blood cell life	mustard greens, turnip greens, chard, sunflower seeds, almonds, spinach, collard greens, parsley, kale, papaya, olives, bell pepper, brussels sprouts, kiwifruit, tomato, blueberries, broccoli
Vitamin K	Deficiency in pregnant women and newborns common	Bleeding disorders	spinach, brussels sprouts, swiss chard, green beans, asparagus, broccoli, kale, mustard greens, green peas, carrots.
Zinc	68% of diets deficient	Acne, amnesia, apathy, brittle nails, delayed sexual maturity, depression, diarrhea, eczema, fatigue, growth impairment, hair loss, high cholesterol levels, immune impairment, impotence, irritability, lethargy, loss of appetite, loss of sense of taste, low stomach acid, male infertility, memory impairment, night blindness, paranoia, white spots on nails, wound healing impairment	calf's liver, crimini mushrooms, spinach, sea vegetables, basil, thyme, spinach, pumpkin seeds, yeast, beef, lamb, beef, lamb, summer squash, asparagus, venison, chard, collard greens, miso, shrimp, maple syrup, broccoli, peas, yogurt, pumpkin seeds, sesame seeds, mustard greens

Source: see Resources section for list of sources   *RDA = Recommended Daily Allowance

Chapter 8
Changing your mind

Many people worry that they'll "change" after surgery. They worry they might become the type of person they don't like. Or their loved ones worry they'll see unpleasant personality changes once the weight is gone after bariatric surgery. Is this really something you need to worry about? Are you afraid of change? Will you change after surgery?

Yes, you are going to change. But change is good!

Change is part of the process — a very important part of your weight loss journey. Change is essential. Without change, bariatric surgery cannot work. But how you change is completely up to you. Deliberate and positive change is the type of change we are striving for. Use your bariatric surgery as your opportunity to make the changes you want to see in your life.

- Are you tired of hiding behind your weight?

- Do you want to be more outgoing and adventurous?

- Do you want to get more involved in your community and make new friends?

- Do you want to feel more secure emotionally, financially, spiritually and intellectually?

- Do you want to be more confident in the person you are so you can embrace the attitude and personality you've been hiding for too long?

- Do you want your relationships to be stronger, happier and more fun?

- Do you want to become more in tune with your spiritual self?

- Do you want to travel more?

- Do you want to dance and play?

- Do you want to get out of debt and stop worrying about money?

- Do you want to go back to school or change careers?

- What else do you want to change?

At what other time in your life have you ever had the opportunity to make the changes you've been resisting all along? Weight loss surgery is a turning point in your life; it is a springboard for creating change. Nothing is holding you back now — not your weight, not your self-esteem, not your health.

You have made the decision to have bariatric surgery. You've decided to change your relationship with food. You've decided to be more active and learn to love exercise and make it a part of your life. You've made the decision to improve the wonderful person you already are. These decisions are the type of decisions made by a person who wants to see extraordinary positive change in their life.

This is a time for celebration and excitement. This is a time to embrace change and seek it out.

I challenge you to make a list of all the things you have ever dreamed of achieving in your life. Make it a list that's lofty and without limits. Dream the biggest dreams you can think of and write them down. Then take a few things off that big list and start working on them one by one. Share your goals with loved ones and keep a journal to track your progress.

Comprehensive Holistic Wellness Plan

A few months after my surgery I participated in a group therapy session with other weight loss surgery patients. This session was conducted by Dr. Gerard Williams in Flint, Michigan, a neuropsychologist who has worked with bariatric patients for over 20 years. One small part of that therapy session was to create a Comprehensive Holistic Wellness Plan.

Of all the things I learned in that 10-week therapy session, this Wellness Plan has had the greatest impact on my life. (*Thank you, Dr. Williams!*)

Weight loss surgery throws you into the middle of some very big life changes. I knew these changes were coming and I was not willing to just let change happen in my life. I'm a bit of a control freak (yes, I'm working on that), so I wanted to make sure the changes I was going to make took me to the place I envisioned for my future.

Being the "Googlehead" that I am had to go find definitions for each of the words in the title of this big scary life plan. Comprehensive Holistic Wellness Plan. Seeing the definitions really helped to get a clear picture of what this thing is all about.

Comprehensive — Of large scope; covering or involving much; inclusive; covering completely or broadly; extensive understanding.

Holistic — Emphasizing the importance of the whole and the interdependence of its parts. Emphasizing the organic or functional relation between parts and the whole.

Wellness — The quality or state of being healthy in body and mind, especially as the result of deliberate effort.

Plan — A scheme or method of acting, doing, proceeding worked out beforehand for the accomplishment of an objective.

As part of this Wellness Plan, I set some very specific goals — not just weight loss specific goals, but goals that touched all areas of my life. I wanted a healthy life and I knew that my health is not measured only about a number on the bathroom scale. A healthy life is about the big picture and includes a lot more than just physical health.

These life goals have plans that won't be achieved in a month or year or two years - these are goals that I plan to steadily work toward for many years to come. My plan includes:

- Physical health
- Spiritual health
- Financial health
- Vocational health
- Intellectual health
- Emotional health
- Relationships health
- Character health

I'm still working on these changes. I'm continually revisiting the detailed plans and adjusting my tasks as I work toward the change I want to see. Some of these goals have projections that go five or ten years into the future. It's a difficult process that takes a lot of work and dedication but I'm glad I started working on these goals early in my journey.

By setting specific goals for what you want to achieve in your life, you have control over the changes that will take place after your surgery (or at anytime in your life!).

You are definitely going to change after surgery and for many people it become the negative change that I eluded to at the beginning of this chapter. So you can either let change happen randomly or negatively, or you can take charge of the changes that will happen as you begin this new chapter of your life and create positive change in your life.

The mental stuff

It wasn't long after my weight loss surgery when I realized that this journey to a healthier me has very little to do with the physical surgery. Yes, the newly formed stomach pouch and rerouted digestive tract put me on the path to losing weight and I never could have achieved the success I have seen without the surgery. But I soon realized that most of the work of this surgery is about the "mental stuff."

I believe that weight loss surgery journey is only about 10% the physical surgery and all the rest is:

- Figuring out how to have a healthy relationship with food

- Understanding that food was not designed to be used as an emotional companion and finding a way to deal with your emotions without food

- Learning to love yourself enough to make the healthy choices in your life

- Discovering why you became obese in the first place and fixing that problem so it can never become an excuse for regaining weight

I don't mean to diminish the importance of the surgery. That is not the intent here. Without that 10% portion of the surgery, it is simply not possible to achieve the other 90% — so the surgery is an essential part of the whole. But remember that you can't rely completely on the surgery. You must do the hardest parts on your own.

A healthy relationship with food

God created us with taste buds. And to me, that means we are designed to enjoy the taste of food — the full spectrum of food. We are meant to savor the flavors of food and experience all the different tastes and textures that were created for us to enjoy.

Unfortunately, many of us obese folks have abused the joy of food for so long that we now think of food as the enemy. Food made us fat, so it must be evil, right? No! Food is not evil — food is neither good nor bad — food is just food. It is your lack of respect for food that caused you to overeat and gain weight. How long have you been relying on food to fill a void in your emotional life? It has to stop!

Many of us after WLS develop hatred toward food. We believe that food is what caused our obesity so it's evil and all "bad" food must be avoided forever. But rather than trying to learn how to "hate" food, or think of it as mere fuel, I think it's more important to learn how to have a healthy relationship with food. A relationship that nourishes your body and provides the important vitamins and minerals needed for survival, but also allows you to enjoy the food you eat without using it as an emotional crutch, shield or weapon.

Unfortunately, for many of us we have developed an unhealthy relationship with food throughout our lives and use it for something other than what it was intended. Food was never supposed to hide emotion or make us feel better when we're stressed or angry or sad. And teaching our minds to have a different view of food, of respecting it and enjoying it for what it is — that's where the big learning curve comes into play after surgery.

As you begin developing this healthy relationship with food, you're now faced with the question of how to handle the emotions you have always buried with food. Instead of trying to bury your "sadness with chocolate cake," you need to learn how to resolve the sadness and work through those emotions in a different, more productive way. Sometimes you just need to sit with your emotions and allow yourself to actually feel them. It's okay to be sad (or angry or happy or stressed) and it's okay to allow yourself to feel those feelings. You don't need to hide those feelings or channel them into some other new hobby or distraction. Emotions are normal — go ahead, feel them.

You also need to learn about moderation. I once said: "I can't live the rest of my life without lemon meringue pie on Thanksgiving." So if I plan to have pie on Thanksgiving, I need to learn how to control myself enough to have a small slice of pie instead of three slices — or one plate of food on Thanksgiving instead of going back three or four times. Moderation needs to be factored into the process of that healthy relationship with food too.

But how do you develop this new relationship and not allow food to remain the emotional companion it's been for so many years? How do you learn about moderation without letting compulsive overeating take control of your good intentions? It's all possible. But it takes a lot of hard work. The battle against emotional eating is one that must be fought with the right weapons. If you have an arsenal filled with all the right weapons and learn how to use them when they're needed — you have come a long way toward developing that healthy relationship with food.

The Battle Against Emotional Eating:
Arming yourself with the weapons you need to win the fight

Emotional eating is a battle you'll fight every day for the rest of your life. You can't make it go away; instead you have to learn how to manage it. Losing weight doesn't fix it, getting healthy or exercising a lot doesn't eliminate the behavior, it's a habit you must confront on an intellectual level. Here are some strategies to help you cope with emotions without turning to food.

In this section I'll give you writing assignments that will help you build your arsenal of weapons to help you battle emotional eating. So grab a journal and prepare to work through this section with pen in hand.

Know that it's okay to have emotions. Emotions are a perfectly natural part of who we are as humans. But that doesn't mean we like feeling sad or stressed or overextended. But when we experience an unpleasant emotion, we don't need to bury it or try to get rid of it, which is what we do when we respond to negative emotions by eating.

Instead try this: Sit quietly for a moment and acknowledge your emotions. If you're angry, then be angry. If you're sad, then be sad. If you're happy, just be happy. You don't need food to acknowledge those emotions; you need to recognize the feeling, accept it and move on with your day.

For so many years we've allowed food to keep us safe from the emotions we don't want to face; always keeping our back to those ugly emotions. But now it's time to turn around and look those emotions square in the face and confront them. No more running away, not more hiding or ignoring the feelings you have. It's time to allow emotion into your life without the compulsive need to bury it with food.

Name your emotions

Make a list of as many different emotions as you can think of. List everything you can think of, even if you don't typically feel those emotions. This step will help to identify all the different possible combinations of emotional eating. I've started a list for you in the sidebar.

Know your emotional triggers

It's essential to understand which of your emotions will cause you to reach for food. And more importantly, which triggers get out of control the fastest. Perhaps you are a stress eater but you are avoid food when you're angry. Or maybe stress isn't a problem for you but when you're bored you turn to food. Do you treat the family to ice cream sundaes when something good happens and you want to celebrate?

Think about times when you've turned to food in an emotional situation. What were you feeling in each of these situations? Think about your list and write it all down. Look at every emotion you wrote down in the previous step and determine if that emotion causes you to reach for food.

Take the time to explore the reasons behind why certain emotions make you eat but others don't. This is a process, so don't rush it. Work in small chunks and keep coming back to this list to continue exploring your emotions on paper. Thinking about it is fine, but writing it down makes those thoughts real so it's important to literally use pen and paper in this exercise.

Make a list of your trigger foods

What foods do you turn to when you are experiencing strong emotions (i.e.: sweets, salty snacks, alcohol, healthy foods in unhealthy amounts)? You might think you already know the answers, but the reality might surprise you. Turn back to that list of the times you experienced emotional eating. What did you eat? Where did you get the food? Where you alone or with a group? Did you recognize that you were out of control? What made you stop?

Name Your Emotions

- Playfulness
- Loneliness
- Obligation
- Envy
- Love
- Remorse
- Contempt
- Frugality
- Sadness
- Surprise
- Feat
- Anxiety
- Joy
- Disappointed
- Trust
- Depression
- Agitation
- Hurt
- Stress
- Guilt
- Happy
- Despair
- Pride
- Affection
- Shame
- Weariness
- Doubt
- Boredom
- Anticipation
- Irritation
- Sorrow
- Excitement
- Worry
- Grief
- Resentment
- Entitlement
- Craving
- Passion
- Weariness

Write these foods down and begin to explore the reasons behind why you reach for different types of foods in different situations. Make a physical list in your journal so you can refer back to it later. This exercise can help you recognize the behavior when you're emotionally eating. But remember that not every emotion has the same trigger foods. Perhaps when you're under stress you reach for sweet treats but when you're angry you go for alcohol or salty snacks. For instance, when I'm angry I know that I reach for chocolate but when I'm bored, I go for salty snacks instead. By exploring the details of each individual emotion, you will have a clearer picture of which battles you must fight when the emotion creeps up.

Make the call

As you work through the list of emotions and learn to identify your triggers, you'll learn how to recognize the warning signs of emotional eating before it gets out of control. When you find that you are in the midst of eating because of your emotions, you must take the first step toward stopping that behavior. It takes practice, so you need to be patient with yourself. Begin with this easy first step:

Say out loud: "I'm not hungry, I'm emotional."

Thinking it to yourself doesn't work, you have to say it out loud; hear it spoken and acknowledge that the action you're about to take is emotion-based and not hunger-based. This first step might not actually stop you from eating whatever food you're about to put in your mouth. But it's an important step in the learning process.

Being able to identify the emotion early is essential also. Learn to recognize when strong emotional situations are about to arise and what the warning signs are. For example, if long hours at work and no scheduled down time make you feel resentful toward your job and others in your life and makes you reach for a candy bar - then make a plan that gives you the time you need to de-stress. By having a strategy you are actively acknowledging your emotions and learning how to live with those emotions in a healthy manner.

Keep an emotional journal

Writing down your daily feelings will help you learn how to "make the call" and begin to recognize the steps leading up to certain emotions. This journal doesn't need to be complicated, simply spend five minutes a day writing down how you felt at different times throughout the day. Did you let food sooth your emotions? Did you allow food to be a companion or a celebrant in your life? Record those instances in your journaling. Over time you'll be able to identify any patterns that might need adjusting.

Stock your Emotional Eating Arsenal

Now that you have identified the problem, it's time to explore the solution. You need an arsenal that is well stocked and at the ready when you need it. The right weapon — or tool — is essential. If you need to drive a nail, a toolbox filled with screwdrivers won't do you any good. In your Emotional Eating Arsenal you'll have lists of techniques to employ and activities to do instead of eating. And yes, I mean literal lists on real paper written with an actual pen. Tangible weapons are essential to this process, so do the work necessary to build your arsenal. You wouldn't send a soldier into battle with a gun and tank that's just a figment of their imagination, right? So neither should you go into battle against emotional eating with just an "idea" of what you might do in case you reach for food when you shouldn't.

Find something else to do

If you eat when you're bored, find a hobby that occupies your hands (knitting, scrapbooking, gardening). If you eat when you're happy, figure out how to release that joyous energy in a positive way (turn the radio up loud and dance around the house with the kids). If you eat when you're angry, find a way to get the aggression out (kickboxing, weight lifting, scrubbing toilets). Make a list of ideas - this list becomes an important weapon. By creating this list of ideas, when you're in the midst of an emotional rant you don't have to be responsible for thinking clearly to find something to release the emotions, just refer to the list in your arsenal and pick something.

Phone-a-Friend

When you're faced with emotion and find yourself standing in front of an open refrigerator, you know you're weak. Lean on someone you trust and who will listen. Pick up the phone, send an email, get on Facebook or join a chat room. Start writing a list of all the friends and family members you can count on in this situation — include their phone number, email address or screen name. As you build the list of your circle of friends, you will find others who struggle with the same things you do. Today you'll be the one doing the leaning — but next week, you might be the one to give support to someone else.

As GI Joe says: Knowing is half the battle

As you work through this process there will be times when you know you're eating for emotional reasons rather than hunger. And we all know that many times emotions are much more powerful than the logical brain — quite frankly, sometimes emotions get the upper hand.

But knowing or recognizing that you're in the midst of an emotional eating binge is an important step. Remember back when you wouldn't think twice about eating for whatever reason you felt like eating? Working toward awareness is a huge step in the right direction. Over time, you'll grow stronger and better able to handle your emotions in a healthier way.

Forgive Yourself. Mistakes happen

No matter how hard we try, emotional eating is going to happen. When it does, don't let guilt plague you and make it even worse. We're not allowed to indulge in guilt-eating to make up for the emotional-eating! Instead, acknowledge that you made a mistake forgive yourself and move on. Don't dwell on it. Just make the very next step, the very next meal or snack...the right choice.

What not to do

Very often I hear people give advice to just replace the "bad food" with a healthier choice. Instead of eating chocolate cake when you're sad, reach for carrot sticks instead. Yeah right! That's why this advice can be dangerous — the habit of eating for emotional reasons is still there. It's important to address the emotions involved in your life and how you manage those emotions — once you are able to live with the emotion and stop trying to bury it or hide it or sooth it, your behaviors will reflect this healthier mental state.

Your Emotional Eating Arsenal

Emotions are OK	*Sit quietly for a moment and acknowledge your emotions*
Say it Out Loud	*I'm not hungry. I'm emotional*
Emotional Triggers	*Explore reasons behind why certain emotions make you eat*
Eating Triggers	*What foods do you turn to? Make a list for each emotion*
Make the Call	*Recognize the warning signs before it gets out of control*
Emotional Journal	*Spend 5 minutes a day writing down how you felt today*
Activity List	*Create a list of activities to do instead of eating*
Phone-a-Friend	*List Lean on someone you trust and who will listen*
Awareness	*Know when you're eating out of emotions rather than hunger*
Mistake Strategy	*Acknowledge when you make a mistake, forgive yourself & move on*

Loving yourself enough

As a child I was taught not to let others put me down or talk to me in a negative way, but sometimes the person attacking my own self-worth and criticizing my efforts toward success is me! The words you use in your minds can become a very powerful tool — either negative or positive. Negative self-talk has a way of becoming a self-fulfilling prophecy and the mean words you say to yourself start to become the reality you don't want to live.

For instance when you feel defeated and start complaining that the challenge you face is "too hard" or "impossible" — then you will stop looking for ways to solve the problem or you'll merely give up on the challenge and accept defeat. If you keep telling yourself you're a "slow loser" after WLS — even when, in reality, you probably aren't a slow loser — you'll start doing things that might sabotage your success like eating poorly or skipping workouts.

Negative self-talk can also increase stress levels and create anxiety within your mind and body. Increased stress levels produce a hormone called cortisol. Increased levels of cortisol have been shown to influence weight gain, memory problems, insulin resistance and even Type 2 Diabetes. If negative self-talk about your weight is causing your increased stress then that self-fulfilling prophecy may have some basis in basic biology too.

Recognizing negative self-talk is the essential first step in the process of stopping it. Some examples of negative self-talk include:

- Belittling yourself for minor missteps or mistakes

- Being critical of your body, weight loss attempts or self-worth

- Saying negative things about yourself to family, friends, or strangers

- Brushing off compliments from other with a negative reply (just say thank you!)

- Doubting your abilities, skills, or expertise

- Giving up in the face of a difficult challenge

Once you are quickly able to identify negative self-talk, you need stop the thought process immediately. A psychologist once taught me a technique called Thought Stopping — which literally means to scream STOP! as loud as you can inside your head. This will interrupt the pattern of negative thoughts and let your brain sit up and take notice of what new message you are about to give it. Once you have the attention of your brain, you can give it something positive to gnaw on for a while.

But you can't expect to think up a bunch of positive self-talk phrases at a moment's notice right after you use Thought Stopping. You need to have a list of positive self-talk phrases at the ready for those moments of distress.

Start a Love List

Keeping a list of positive accomplishments in your journal (or taped to your refrigerator) is the only way to quickly turn negative self-talk into positive. Your Wow Moment list is a great starting point and you can add to that list with other amazing accomplishments, skills, and triumphs you have achieved. This list can become your Love List — all the things you love about yourself and all the things you are great at and worked hard to accomplish.

Once you get this Love List created, keep adding to it as you do new and amazing things. And keep a copy of it close at hand — whether you carry your journal around with you, or create a summary of the list and keep it on a card in your wallet, whatever it takes to keep the list handy when you need to put a stop to the negative thoughts.

The most important first step in turning negative self-talk into positive self-talk is to simply stop saying, "I can't" and start saying, "I going to try..."

Your self-talk is directly related to your self-worth and self-esteem. When you love yourself enough to say kind things to yourself, you are well on your way to a healthier life.

Throughout this journey to a healthier you, it is important that you love yourself enough to do what is right and healthy for your body every day for the rest of your life. That includes the physical stuff like making healthy choices in the foods you eat, taking your required vitamins, drinking enough water and getting the right amount of exercise. But it also included the mental stuff too — like getting a handle on emotional eating, learning why you allowed yourself to become morbidly obese in the first place and finding a way to maintain good self-esteem.

Loving yourself enough should also include the other areas of your health like your spiritual health, financial health, intellectual health and others.

Some ways to learn how to love yourself more:

- Make a Love List of everything you love (or like) about yourself
- Ask family and friends to contribute their own Love List about you
- Find one thing about yourself each day that you're proud of and add it to your Love List
- Use positive daily affirmations to reinforce your love
- Be kind to yourself
- Indulge in self-pampering regularly
- When someone gives you a compliment, write it on your Love List
- Forgive yourself - for past self-hatred, for self-doubt, for mistakes or shortcomings or anything else weighing on your mind
- Believe in yourself and understand that you are worthy of love

This whole self-love thing sounds pretty easy on paper. But I know, from experience, that the actual work it takes to turn self-loathing (or even just self-disinterest) into self-love is pretty difficult and takes a lot of hard work. Even though I've only been working on this process since my surgery, I've got a long way to go to be all the way to true self-love — but each day I get a little bit closer. I think this is going to be a lifelong process.

You'll spend hours with your emotional journal and shed lots of tears as you make the journey to self-discovery. It's hard to put yourself first for a change, but it's something we all have to do if we want to enjoy a healthy and happy life. All the hard work, time and energy are worth it though.

Putting Yourself First

As obese people, especially us women, we tend to put ourselves last on the list of priorities. We always want to take care of everyone else in our lives and make sure we don't create any waves or hurt anyone else's feelings. We always put ourselves at the bottom of the list and we tolerate it when others do the same. It's a common trait of morbidly obese people.

So how do we fix that bad habit? Practice and commitment.

When I had my weight loss surgery I made a commitment to myself for the first year post-op. I decided that I was going to be very selfish and put myself first. As a single woman, I took myself off the dating market for a full year and

I also warned my family members that they might be hearing "no" from me a bit more often than they cared for. I dedicated those first 12 months — a full 365 days — to my physical and emotional health. It's one of the best decisions I made. After that first year I opened up a little bit more, but there are still times when I recognize that I need to take a step back from pleasing others and take the time to pamper myself.

When you are taking care of yourself - when you are healthy and happy — you are better equipped both physically and emotionally to take care of those around you. Remember that instruction from your last airline trip? Place the oxygen mask over your own face before you attempt to help those around you. What good would you be to your family members if you're too sick, stressed or overwhelmed to even take care of yourself?

Do you catch yourself saying things like: "I'm too busy to pack a lunch so I just grab something fast." or "I try to remember to take my vitamins, but things are always crazy around here." Those are the types of statements that indicate you aren't putting yourself first.

Take the time for a bit of meal planning at the beginning of the week so you have healthy meal choices ready later in the week when things get busy. Set a timer on your mobile phone to remind you to take your vitamins. Get into the habit of carrying a bottle of water with you everywhere you go so you meet your water intake goals. Schedule exercise into your day and invite the family to tag along. Make a date with yourself each week to do something that rejuvenates your soul. Take two minutes each morning to slather on yummy smelling body lotion. All these little things add up to a healthy and balanced life filled with self-love.

Many years ago I got into the habit of doing something for myself once a week that I completely enjoyed. In the summer it might be spending a Saturday afternoon reading a book at the beach with my toes tucked into the hot sand. In the winter I enjoy going to a local coffeehouse and listening to the live acoustic music they host each Friday night. In the early fall I love walking along the trails enjoying the autumn colors of Michigan and soaking up some of God's creation. Or maybe it's an occasional pajama day where I veg in front of the television with a stack of rented movies.

Not matter what luxury I decide to indulge in for the week, I do it completely guilt-free and I give myself permission to put all the stresses of life on hold for those few hours. Try it yourself, you'll fall in love with the concept.

The problem with putting yourself first is that those around you will not be happy about the change. You'll be faced with resistance but you need to stand strong in this decision. When we make such a drastic change in our lives with weight loss surgery and we're changing everything about how we act and what we do - we have to take the plunge and have faith that we'll be better for the changes and selfishness.

No matter how much your family thinks they understand what you're going through, I have found that they simply cannot comprehend it all. I know this because I was one of those people who thought I understood what post-op life was going to be like.

Can Non-WLS Folks Understand Us?

Before I had surgery I thought I understood what my sister and mother had gone through in their WLS journey. They ate smaller meals and had to limit the "bad food" and lost weight. It was just a strict diet, right?

I learned a bit more as I was going through the research phase for my own surgery. I learned more about the mental and emotional side of the surgery and all the changes I would need to make. I read about the struggles other post-ops experienced and in my mind knew the "right" answers to all those questions about head hunger and food addiction and no longer being able to use food as a comfort or companion. I felt that I had a very good understanding of life after surgery. I felt prepared. I knew there were struggles to be faced. I also knew that I was strong enough to face them.

But when I look back to my understanding before surgery of those struggles I realize I knew very little about what was about to come. I knew so little about what I would really be facing and all the stuff that can only be understood after you are living the life and standing in the trenches of the battle for your health.

I spent almost a year and a half researching this surgery and lifestyle changes I'd need to make. I watched my sister and mother through their surgeries for five years before my surgery. Yet I was surprised at the magnitude of the struggle that I was expected to face.

Can anyone really get it unless they've walked in our shoes and had to live through the struggle themselves? Can our family members understand? Can our friends comprehend? Is there a way to explain it to them that would help them understand better? If there is, I haven't found a way.

My best friend, a non-WLS person, once said to me: "What's the big deal? You had surgery months ago, aren't you healed yet?"

Yes, my surgical wounds had healed and my body was functioning like it should have been. But I was still in the trenches of the emotional turmoil that goes along with the life changes I was making. My work was just beginning but my friend didn't understand that I needed to shed the mentality of obesity and learn a new way of thinking about food and about myself. My friend understands me better now that I've had a chance to explain the changes I was working on. But that conversation made me realize how little non-WLS people really understand about us, even if they support us with every fiber of their being.

Oh sure, I could treat this process as "just a strict diet" and continue eating the same food I used to eat, just in smaller portions. I could stop worrying so much about the changes I want to make to my emotional health or the other areas of my life I want to improve. But if I don't deal with the mental aspect of what landed me at obesity's doorstep, I'm only putting myself at risk for regaining the weight and falling back into bad habits.

Do I really want to go back to being the person who stops at Domino's after work to pick up dinner — and eats the majority of a pizza alone? No. Do I want to go back to being the person who is bored at home on a Sunday morning so bakes a cake and eats a third of it before work on Monday? No. I don't want food to be a controlling force in my life. I don't want food to be the first thing I think of when I'm trying to find something to occupy my time. I don't want my vacations to be planned around where we'll eat.

So to make those physical changes to my body and emotional changes to my mind's way of thinking about food — it's necessary to change every aspect of my life.

I want to deal with the emotions I feel. I want to figure out some alternative way of dealing with my boredom, laziness, happiness, sadness or whatever other emotion that causes people to eat instead of face the emotion and manage it without food. And the only way I can do that is to face those demons head on and fight them to the death.

But for someone who doesn't struggle with those demons, they probably won't ever get it, will they?

I want my life to be a certain way. And in order to achieve that I have to work really hard to make the changes I want to see. What other time in my life will I ever have the perfect opportunity to get healthy in all areas of my life?

This journey is more than just a strict diet. It's about getting in touch with who I am and what I'm about. It's about figuring out how to love myself, despite my flaws, while still working to fix as many of those flaws as I can. I'm not sure anyone can really understand what that's like until they've gone through it themselves.

So I guess that means that when the surgeon wheels us into the operating room, we need to ask him to implant some extra patience while he's in there. We'll get frustrated with our friends and family members (or complete strangers) who don't understand what we're going through, but we have to pile on the patience and kindheartedness for their lack of understanding.

Working toward Normal

In the weeks and months after weight loss surgery you'll find that your whole world revolves around the surgery and the changes you are making. This is normal. In fact, this is a very good thing and will help you be more successful in the long term as you make permanent changes in your life.

Lynnda and Toni from BariatricTV.com's online television webisodes have termed the phrase "surgical freaks" when describing us post-op folks. I love the term! They define freak as someone with a strange deviation from the norm or someone who spends more than the usual time devoted to an activity or interest. So by definition, we are freaks — our guts have been rearranged and life becomes devoted to the whole process of WLS and changing our lives to become healthier. I'm a Surgical Freak!

But after a while you start to resent your differences. In fact, I once said that I was tired of hearing myself think about weight loss surgery and I just needed a break from myself. (That lasted about a minute!) The ultimate goal with having surgery, for me, was to be normal.

Remember at the beginning of the book when I mentioned a list of reasons I wanted to have surgery? Below is that list — notice I never focused on the actual weight I wanted to be, just the way I wanted to feel about myself.

- When I go to the mall to shop for a new outfit, I want to be able to shop at a normal store and find a variety of outfits to choose from. Not a plus size shop, not a skinny-minny shop, just a normal old store.

- When I go to a restaurant I want to eat off the menu and have a portion that is normal. Not a huge, oversized portion that would feed three people and not a tiny WLS portion that I ate in the early months post-op, I want to eat a normal size portion.

- When I'm in a photo of a group of people, I want to be a normal size. I don't want to be the fattest person and don't need to be the smallest person either. But I just want to blend in and look normal.

- When I go to the gym I want to fit in with the rest of the athletic people. I don't want to be the fat chick who's trying too hard and I don't want to be the hot chick who is only there to pick up guys. I just want to feel like I fit in, that I'm normal.

- When I think about food I want to feel normal. Meal planning, counting calories, counting protein grams, making sure I get all my water and vitamins, it's an obsession. I want it all to be second nature. I don't want to be so focused on food and my daily schedule. I just want to feel normal with my whole daily eating routine.

For many months after surgery you will literally feel like a freak of nature. Your world revolves around this major change in your lifestyle. You're focused on goals and eating the right foods and establishing new routines. You'll hope that one day you arrive at a place where my surgery is not the main focus of life. It'll always be there, but it won't always to be the first thing you think of in the morning and the last thing on your mind before bed. One day you'll somehow arrive at normal — or at least in the suburbs of normal.

So when you start to feel a bit freakish, please remember that one day you'll do something in the midst of your daily routine and you'll realize you just brushed elbows with normal.

Why am I Fat?

First, let me just say that I know there are many people who battle obesity that have medical conditions that contributed to uncontrolled weight gain. But this is rarer than we'd like to believe. Often a medical condition plays a minor role in obesity but gets the majority of the blame. If you are one of the rare people who truly gained weight because of a medical problem, then this next part is not for you.

Most cases of morbid obesity are based in some type of emotional difficulty which manifests itself in physical behaviors, but doctors only give dieting advice based the physical behavior and rarely address the emotional issues at the core of the problem.

Even when you undergo serious, life-altering bariatric surgery, you are often not educated in how to make the emotional changes necessary to become long-term success stories. Surgery to alter your stomach and cause you to eat less food will not correct the problem of eating to bury emotion or fill a void in your life or respond to a compulsion where you have little control. Until you dig into your mind and soul to find the root cause of your obesity and figure out a way to fix it, you'll never truly conquer morbid obesity.

In my personal opinion, the rate of post-op weight regain is a direct result of patients not facing the cause of their own individual obesity and finding a way to overcome those issues. Surgeons do the operation on your stomach; they don't do surgery on your brain. All the psychological work that needs to be done is the responsibility of the patient - nobody can make the emotional changes except you. And it's the hardest part of this whole process.

Yes, you read that right. The mental part of this healthy journey is the hardest part and it takes the most amount of work. Figuring out the reason you became morbidly obese in the first place is the first step to recovery from the disease of obesity. But how do you figure out why you got fat? Isn't it just that I loved food and ate too much of it? Isn't that fixed with surgery anyway? Can my surgeon tell me why I'm fat?

No. Unfortunately there's no simple solution to this puzzle. None of us will have the same reason for our obesity. Our surgeon can't tell us why. A psychologist can help you discover the answer, but nobody can uncover the truth except you.

Luckily you already know which reason is not the root of your obesity: the fact that you just enjoyed food and liked to eat — that's not the reason. Neither is the notion that your parents didn't teach you how to eat healthy. Those are behaviors that caused obesity. But remember that your behaviors are based in emotion. So you have to dig deeper than the behavior and figure out the reason why you behaved that way. Why did you have a love affair with food? What was missing in your life that caused you to turn to food for companionship? Or what were you trying to hid that food could disguise?

So you first must identify the behavior that led to morbid obesity, then identify the emotions or psychological reasons you allowed that behavior to become so out of control that you gained enough weight that it required you to have bariatric surgery.

I'm not trying to be harsh or critical in being so direct about this part of the journey. But please understand that unless we figure out this part there is no way that we can successfully maintain a healthy lifestyle or avoid weight regain. This journey of discovery can't be rushed, of course, and it might take you years to discover the whole answer. But as long as you're working on it little by little and realize that until you are healthy on a psychological level, the physical health can never follow.

I had to do the hard work to figure it out for myself (thankfully, with some help from a therapist) and then once I figured it out, I had to dig deeper and find out what else I was using as a crutch for my obesity.

I'm thankful that I learned my reason early in my WLS journey. But even once I had the word for why I let myself get fat, I still had a lot of work to do when digging to the core of that reason. By no means am I all the way there. I've got a long way to go and I'm learning new things about myself all the time.

Entitlement. That's my reason. I would use excuses like: "I worked hard this week, I deserve to order a pizza for dinner" or "I've been so good on my diet, I deserve a treat." But then I had to discover what was at the core of that entitled thinking. Through a lot of journaling, soul-searching, tears, and enlightenment, I have been able to uncover, layer-by-layer where that sense of entitlement came from. Much of it was based in a cash-strapped childhood, a very strict private college experience, an early career in a job with too many rules, and I'm sure that my naturally rebellious nature probably contributed, as well. I won't go into the details - because it's not very exciting - but I understand how important this process is to my success in concurring obesity and I'm still doing the work necessary to be as healthy as I can be.

Now whenever I catch myself trying to justify a poor food choice or unhealthy behavior with the word "deserve" — I know that's the keyword in recognizing I'm allowing the entitlement to creep back into my life.

I hope that you will also find your reason and learn how to manage it. A therapist can help you with the process and I highly recommend you talk to someone trained in working with bariatric patients.

Self-Doubt

Before any of us undergo weight loss surgery we have spent years and years trying to lose weight through diet and exercise alone. Maybe some of us could lose weight, but not keep it off. Maybe some, like me, couldn't lose weight at all, no matter how hard they tried. Or maybe some would lose a few pounds, got discouraged and would give up and go back to old habits.

The cycle of failed diet after failed diet is frustrating and discouraging and begins to wear on your self-esteem and causes self-doubt to move in and take up residency. Nobody likes to fail. And when we have faced so much failure in our weight loss attempts over so many years, is it any surprise that we approach weight loss surgery with that load of self-doubt still weighing heavy on our hearts?

We want to have faith and believe that weight loss surgery is going to work for us. But it's hard to believe that we'll finally lose the excess weight and get healthy for good, especially when all the other times we believed the same thing, we were handed Failure on a silver platter.

It doesn't matter how excited you are about your surgery or how convinced that the scientific studies are true when they tell you it's going to work — in the back of your mind there's this little seed of doubt. Some acknowledge it openly and talk about it and ask questions about it. Some are too afraid to realize it's there and try to ignore it. But there are a few who recognize the doubt, face it, confront it and beat it into submission. Self-doubt is a powerful emotion. It's also a powerful motivator.

Self-doubt can be a motivator in two ways. First, it can set you up for failure and excuses. Second, it can set you up for a battle that you are determined to win no matter the cost. If you let self-doubt live in the back of your mind and act like the on-call excuse, you'll quickly find a way to use it.

I hit a stall, I'm a failure.
I ate a cookie, I'm a failure.
I forgot to take my vitamins, I'm a failure.
I didn't go to the gym today, I'm a failure.

Those self-defeating statements are all based in self-doubt. No, you're not a failure if you stumble or make a mistake or indulge more than you should. It just means you're human and you're living like a normal person. No big deal! Acknowledge the mistake, dust yourself off and move on with the rest of your day. Don't let self-doubt call you names or give you excuses for not doing your best.

Self-doubt can be a motivator for success if you let it. Think of it as the enemy and every day you must fight the battle to win the war. Instead of letting self-doubt creep in and be the catalyst for your failure, let self-doubt become the champion for your success. Instead of those self-defeating statements about failure, try these instead:

I hit a stall. Now I must figure out what needs to be adjusted to make the scale move again.

I ate a cookie. It sure was delicious. Now I need to look at the rest of my day's meal plan and figure out how to adjust my protein intake to compensate for the unplanned carbs and sugar.

I forgot my vitamins today. I need to realize that we all make mistakes and that tomorrow is a new day. I will re-evaluate my vitamin schedule and figure out why I missed doses today and how I can prevent that from happening again.

I didn't go to the gym today. I will check my calendar for the next available day when I can hit the gym to make up for an inactive day or find a way to incorporate more lifestyle activity into my day to make up for a missed workout.

These little adjustments in your attitude about self-doubt play a huge role in your overall success with weight loss surgery. If your attitude is that weight loss surgery is the start of a new way of living your life, rather than just another diet that you're starting (and will fail at) then you will not let self-doubt play a role in your life and attitude. If you are constantly battling your doubts and devising ways to defeat failure, then over time you will grow stronger and stronger in your health and determination to be a success.

Chapter 9
Goals & Triumphs

How do you know if you've achieved a goal unless you first define what success will look like for you. Of course, we all have the goal of losing weight and getting healthy when we have weight loss surgery and I've already talked about a whole-life wellness plan. Both of those types of goals are important as you move through this journey to better health. But what about all the little goals that have to be achieve between now and when you finally cross the finish line on those big life goals? What do you need to accomplish this month, this week, today that will lead you one step closer to accomplishing what you've set out to do?

I believe the little goals, when added all together, are so much more important that the big lofty goals we set because without achieving the small goals — the day-to-day goals — we would never be able to achieve the big ones. The small goals might just seem like a daily or weekly task list. But when you look at that task list as a goal list, you start to see how much work you are accomplishing each day, each week, each month.

When I decided I was going to finish a half-marathon race — 13.1 miles — I didn't just show up on race day to get that goal checked off my list. No. I had a thousand mini-goals between that point of decision and the last step that brought me across the finish line. The first step was signing up for a training program and then buying a good pair of shoes and then showing up on the first day of training and walking that first mile. Each day of my training program had a scheduled walk or cross training assignment — so each one of those daily assignments became a daily goal to achieve that would bring me closer to the ultimate goal of the finish line.

Just like my goal of finishing my college degree, each class assignment, project, tutorial, and final exam brought me one step closer to the degree. But the college degree wasn't the ultimate goal. The degree was just the stepping stone that would take me to a new career path. So while I was burning the midnight oil on studying algebra and learning Photoshop, I was conscious that each class completed would help me be the graphic designer I wanted to be. These two goals were part of my original wellness plan that was spurred by my weight loss surgery – I probably wouldn't have had the courage or ambition to accomplish either one without that first step into the surgeon's office to find out which surgery was right for me.

Weight loss surgery is the beginning of a lifelong venture of achieving goals. We want to be successful in this journey to health, so the first step we must take is defining what success really means. This journey is about our mind, our body, and our soul.

Setting a weight goal

Of course the primary goal of WLS is to lose weight. Too often I see people who are beginning this journey have a very specific, set-in-stone, can't-compromise weight goal and know exactly what the number on the scale will read so they can finally say they are "done." They set their sights on a specific number and live their whole lives around that number.

The number on the scale or the number on the BMI chart or the number on the tag in your pair of jeans — those numbers don't necessarily reflect a true level of health. But unfortunately, the medical community gathers statistics and measure success of patients based on those numbers. That community of professionals includes your surgeon and his/her clinical staff, the scientists who study the numbers and the agencies who keep track of the statistics such as the American Society of Bariatric and Metobolic Surgeons (ASMBS) or the National Institutes of Health (NIH). And don't forget the health insurance industry too. So let's look at what they look at so we understand their statistics of success.

In almost every clinical study I've read about weight loss surgery, the authors consider you a success when you loss 50% of your excess weight. Once you hit the 50% mark, you are added to your surgeon's success list, which means, if you have 100 pounds of excess weight, once you lose 50 pounds, you're a success.

Long term weight loss studies show that RNY patients will lose about 48% to 85% of their excess weight within the first two years post-op and maintain a loss of 53% to 77% at six years post-op.[22]

Since science shows I can expect to lose anywhere from 50% to 85% of my excess weight, why do I automatically assume that I will lose 100% and never look at anything else? Wouldn't it be better to set my weight loss goals based on what the expected outcomes would be based on the surgery type I've chosen? Instead of setting a goal weight on emotion, I had to step outside my own personal comfort zone and use math (oh no!). So, let's look at my weight to do some calculations.

First we must understand what "excess body weight" means. Surgeons primarily use two different methods for calculating ideal body weight. First is the Body Mass Index (BMI) and second is the Metropolitan Life Insurance Weight Chart. The BMI chart is a straight calculation based on height and weight to come up with a number. The Met Life Chart has a ranged of ideal weights based on your gender and body frame size.

The BMI chart has a range of categories for determining if you are normal weight, underweight, overweight, obese or morbidly obese.

BMI	Weight Classification
<18.5	Underweight
18.5–24.9	Normal weight
25–29.9	Overweight
30-34.9	Obesity
35 or 40	Severe obesity
40–44.9	Morbid obesity
≥ 45	Super obese

If you use the BMI scale, you'll notice that the Normal Weight range has a 40 pound variance. For instance, for my height of 5'6" I would need to weight anywhere between 115 and 154 to have a normal weight. If we use the middle of the normal weight range, my ideal weight would be 134 pounds.

Looking at the Met Life Weight Chart, my ideal weight is 130-144 based on a medium frame size. So the center of that range is 137 pounds.

So let's call my ideal weight 135 to make things easier. Which means, starting at 300 pounds before surgery (technically it was 299.4), my total excess body weight is 165 pounds. We know that the scientists expect that we'll lose 50% to 85% of our excess weight in the first two years post-op, and maintain a weight loss of up to 77% - so now it's time to do some math (my least favorite subject!).

Let's calculate what my weight loss would be at each of these important milestone percentages along the weight loss journey.

Pam's Goal Weight Calculations

EBW % Lost	Pounds Lost	Ending Weight
50%	83 lbs.	217 lbs.
77%	127 lbs.	173 lbs.
85%	132 lbs.	168 lbs.
100%	165 lbs.	135 lbs.

What does all this really mean? And how is it supposed to help you set your goal weight?

These numbers mean that when you set a goal weight you need to consider logic and science in your decision rather than just fantasy, pipe dreams, or emotion. It would be a nice thought if I wanted to lose enough weight to fit into my eighth grade softball team uniform, but that goal is not realistic for someone who spent twenty years as a morbidly obese woman. And it's also not realistic to set a weight goal that would have me losing 100% of my excess body weight and completely ignore the statistics of those who went before me on this journey. I'm not saying that 100% isn't possible, but it's not a realistic _first_ goal.

My advice is to set several weight goals and as you achieve each goal, set a new goal to work toward. So your first goal might be to lose 50% of your excess body weight so that you are a statistical success. Then 77% then 85% then finally set your sights on the 100% weight loss goal. Setting incremental goals like this will create momentum in your journey and keep you motivated to continue achieving goals.

There's also the bigger bonus of setting smaller goals and achieving them. Rewards! I love rewards!

Before surgery we would often reward ourselves with food-based rewards - a nice dinner out at our favorite restaurant, an ice cream sundae or a trip to the movies with a big bucket of popcorn. Why did we do silly things like that? But now we know better than to shower ourselves with food rewards. Non-food rewards are so much better anyway.

Achieving your weight goals is not the only time when you should reward yourself. Any goal — big or small — that you set and achieve should always come with a reward. Did you finish your first 5k race? Reward! Did you go a whole month without missing a single day of tracking your food intake? Reward! Did you write in your Emotional Journal five days a week for two months straight? Reward! Set goals and get rewards. Sounds fun, right? I've even provided a list of ideas for your next reward.

Mini–Goals Rewards: *Set small goals that can be achieved in one or two weeks.* Reward Range: Free up to $10

• Movie Tickets	• Lazy guilt-free day	• Spa treatments at home
• Spend time with friends	• Be a kid for an afternoon. Go fly a kite; buy a bunch of balloons and give them away as you go; get a yo-yo and practice silly stunts; go swing on the playground; find a sledding hill or go ice skating.	• Thrift store shopping
• Adopt a pet		• Daylong photography excursion
• New cookbook		• Spend the day playing at your hobby
• New candles		
• Candlelit bubble bath		• Order a "Skinny Latte" from Starbucks and spend the day relaxing with a book
• Buy movie or music from iTunes	• New lipstick or makeup	
• Buy your favorite magazine	• Day at the Beach	• Go hiking or backpacking
	• Road trip, sight-seeing	

Mid-Level Goals Rewards: *Set mid-level goals that can be achieved in a month or two.* Reward Range: $10 - $40

• Workout clothes Running shoes	• Workout clothes Running shoes	• Buy tickets to a play, sporting event or art show
• A massage	• A massage	• Craft supplies
• A manicure/pedicure	• A manicure/pedicure	• Jewelry
• A book, CD or DVD	• A book, CD or DVD	• Take a class
• Dumbbells, medicine ball or resistance bands	• Dumbbells, medicine ball or resistance bands	• Get your car professionally cleaned
• Heart-rate monitor watch	• Heart-rate monitor watch	• Take a "personal" day from work
• Teeth whitening	• Teeth whitening	• Adopt a pet
• Go camping!	• New item of clothing	• Sexy lingerie
• New purse	• Subscribe to a fitness magazine	• Buy yourself flowers
• Candles or home décor`	• Paint a room in your house	• Buy a hammock, set it up and spend the day lazing in the sun
• Day at the beach	• Perfume / Cologne	

Big Goals Rewards: *Set big goals that will take hard work, perseverance, and dedication for the long haul.* Reward Range: $50 and up.

• Vacation or weekend getaway	• Electronic gadget or toy	• New car
• Cruise	• Get a tattoo	• Adopt a pet
• Jewelry (I love bling!)	• Buy tickets to a play, sporting event or art show	• Weekend hobby retreat / trip
• New clothes	• Craft supplies	• Spruce up a room in the house with new décor`
• Makeover	• Hire a personal shopper to help you buy a new wardrobe	• Landscape your house
• Workout equipment	• Buy a new kitchen gadget	• Furniture for the house
• All Day Spa Treatment		
• Hire a maid for a day		

My Success Checklist

Activity Level

☐ Number of workouts this week

☐ Level of intensity of those workouts

☐ How active where you overall

Nutrient & Caloric Intake

☐ Was your eating on track at least 90% of the time?

☐ Did you drink 64oz of water each day?

☐ Did you take all your vitamins and supplements?

Size & Shape

☐ Clothing: is it looser or tighter this week?

☐ Measurements: did your lose or gain inches?

☐ Weight: what did the scale say?

Emotional & Spiritual Health

☐ Did I work on the mental stuff this week?

☐ Did I play this week?

☐ Did I pamper myself?

Wows & Challenges

☐ What Wow Moments, triumphs or goals am I celebrating this week?

☐ What challenges did I face this week?

My Success Score

Devise your own scoring method and rate your success for this week.

Measuring your success without the scale

How do you measure success? Do you let the scale tell you if you're a success or not? Do you let clothing sizes determine your level of success?

Too often we forget that this healthy journey is not about a series of numbers — whether it's our weight or clothing sizes or the number of inches we've lost. There is a whole list of measurements that play into our overall good health. By looking at each one of these different areas of your life, you can see if you are truly doing what's best for your body, your mind, and your soul.

To live a healthy life, you need to be active. And being active isn't only about how much time you spend at the gym on the treadmill; it's also about how intense the workout is and how much more you could be doing. If you've been walking on the treadmill for a while, maybe it's time to see what running is all about.

Being active is also about how much movement you work into your daily routine. You always hear the advice of parking at the back of the lot and walking or taking the steps instead of the elevator or getting up and walking down the hall to speak with a coworker instead of sending an email. All those little bursts of activity count toward your overall level of fitness.

Keeping track of the food you eat and making sure you get enough fluids and all your vitamins — those are essential goals to have each day. Nobody is perfect, which is why I shoot for being on track at least 90% of the time to hit my weekly goals — this journey is about being realistic and striving to do your best.

Of course, your weight and clothing sizes and body measurements need to play some part in measuring your success. But these numbers are not the primary focus; they are just one part of the whole and should receive equal importance with the other categories on the list.

Taking care of your emotional and spiritual health is just as important as your physical health. This includes journaling and working on emotional eating hurdles and your relationship with food, but it also includes finding time to play and to pamper yourself. When I say play, I literally mean play — like you did when you were eight years old. Turn the music high and dance around the house or go play on the monkey bars with the kids at the playground. And take time to indulge in a bit of pampering with a nice bubble bath or a quiet cup of tea after everyone else goes to bed.

The checklist on the opposite page is as a weekly goal worksheet. Each week you review this checklist and record how well you did during the previous days and decide which things you need to work on for the following week. It's easy to get caught up in the hype of what the scale will tell you each day, so having a tool to keep you focused on your overall health is important.

Wow Moments

A Wow Moment is when something happens in your post-op life that literally makes you say "wow!" These moments might be very small observations that happen unexpectedly or they might be huge milestones we've been working toward for months or years.

I highly recommend that you write down your Wow Moments and keep a list. Yes, I mean an actual list written down on paper — don't try to remember these moments because they will be coming too quickly to keep track of them. Even if that moment might seem insignificant when it happens, write it down anyway. This list will be invaluable to you two or three or ten years after your surgery.

The Wow Moments will come fast during the first year or so after surgery but will then taper off the further out you get from surgery. This list of milestones in your early journey will serve as reminder of how far you've come. When the scale stopped moving and I had to adjust my goals and way of thinking about what success meant to me, I got discouraged easily. But having my written list of Wow Moments to look at, helped me remember how amazing this experience is and how many goals I had already achieved.

I could explain it to you all day long, but seeing an actual Wow Moment list is the best explanation. So I'm including some of mine.

Pam's Partial Wow List

- Wow! I can cross my legs and love sitting that way — it's so comfortable!

- Wow! I had to move the driver's seat in my car forward.

- Wow! I bought a size 16 jeans last week!

- Wow! I wore my new swimsuit this weekend. Sat out in front of people with a sheer skirt/wrap on and was completely comfortable in a bathing suit. My self-confidence is getting better for sure.

- Wow! I have a bony butt. My Uncle Phil used to tease me about this when I was a little girl and would sit on his lap, but it's been a long, long time since I've been accused of it.

- Wow! My arms are skinny (well, up to the elbow at least - darn batwings!)

- Wow! My walking group is scheduled to do 7 miles at tomorrow night's training and I'm not worried about it at all. No problem!

- Wow! My best friend said I was looking skinny today.

- Wow! I noticed today that I walk taller and prouder now.

Take Lots of Pictures

Just a couple weeks after my surgery a friend suggested I start taking a photo of my face each day and to continue through the first year after surgery. I took his advice and I'm so glad I did. I set up my tripod in the corner of the living room and each morning I'd snap a quick picture before I left for the day. At the end of the year I put all those pictures together into a video.

Sounds like a fun art project, right? But it's so much more than that!

Dr. Williams, the psychologist who works with my surgeon's office, often reminds us at support group meetings that it takes a while for your mind to catch up with what is going on with your body. He warns it can take up to five years for your brain to truly see the thinner body in the mirror. You have to be patient with yourself and your self-image during this time.

You have to work hard on the process of self-acceptance and one effective way is to take lots of photos of yourself all along the way. Many people report that they can't see the changes in their weight when they look in the mirror, but they can see the changes when they look at pictures. I found that to be true for me too.

The daily face picture project is a big undertaking so you might choose a weekly picture project or even monthly. Take face pictures and full body pictures and profile pictures and even let people snap candid pictures. Whatever you do, don't shy away from the camera!

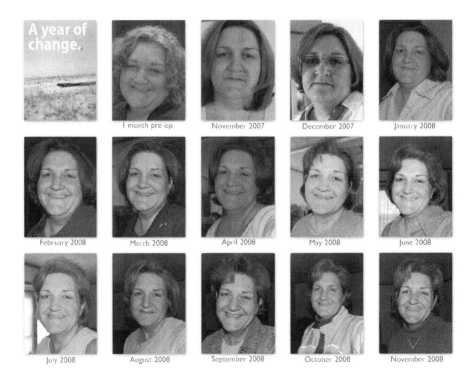

A year of change.

1 month pre-op	November 2007	December 2007	January 2008
February 2008	March 2008	April 2008	May 2008	June 2008
July 2008	August 2008	September 2008	October 2008	November 2008

Chapter 10
When things get hard

This weight loss surgery journey has been the hardest thing I've ever done in my life. And each stage of the process that I'm in always feels like it's the hardest part. I remember when I was just a couple weeks out from surgery and wondering if I'd ever chew solid food again and thinking how hard this whole surgery thing was. Then I arrived at 18 months post-op, the scale had stopped moving and I needed to deal with the mental battle of coming to terms with the fact that my weight loss was finished. Then reactive hypoglycemia set in and I faced another hard part of the journey. Each new battle seemed to be the hardest thing I'd ever done.

This WLS thing is hard! Some parts of it are harder than others, of course. In this section I'll cover some of the issues that we might face on the road ahead. I'll share my own experiences and the information I've gathered from others who have gone before us and how they handled the situation. There is strength in numbers and by all of us going through this together, the battle can be a little bit less hard.

What does it mean to be on track?

Those of us who have chosen WLS as our path to better health understand the terminology associated with the dieting world. When we hear someone talk about being on track, it usually means they are following all the rules and not "cheating" on their diet. We've all been there, we know how that strict dieting lifestyle feels and we understand what that phrase means. But now that I'm living my life as a weight loss surgery patient, my definition of being on track is a bit different than it was when I was trapped inside the yo-yo dieting cycle.

I know that I don't need to be perfect to be on track. My goal is to be on target 90% of the time. And that remaining 10% is just what happens when I'm living my life and I don't allow guilt to creep in for that 10%. In order to be on track, the following must be in place for me:

Love myself enough to take care of my daily needs for better health.

Eat a healthy balance of foods. This includes staying within my calorie range and keeping my macronutrients in line; getting enough fiber and drinking enough water and eating according to my daily schedule to avoid unplanned snacks, grazing or mindless eating. And the only way I'll know if I'm hitting those daily goals is to track my food in my food journal.

Exercise because I care about my overall health. I'm not exercising to lose weight, I'm doing it to improve my heart and lung function, build my lean muscle mass and to be a more healthy person. And it's not just about going to the gym and doing formal workouts, it's about getting out and enjoying life and being more active overall.

Be obsessive about my vitamins and supplements.

Follow the doctor's orders and staying on top of my regular follow up visits with my surgical team.

Be in tune with my body and my emotions and be comfortable with who I am, what I think, how I feel and the direction my life is going.

Be kind to myself. If I fall off track that is not permission to beat myself up. This is not a diet and this is not a race. This is about living my life in a way that is good for my body and makes me happy for the long haul. Be kind. Be happy. Just be.

Breaking a Stall

Weight loss stalls and plateaus are very common after WLS or any type of weight loss program. We didn't gain weight every day over the years and we will not lose weight every day while we're losing. It's frustrating, but it's all part of the process and we just have to be patient and work through these little bumps in the road.

When the scale hasn't moved for a couple weeks or months, this is the perfect time to take a very close look at what you're doing and figure out if you need to make a change. Ask yourself these questions:

- Are you tracking your food intake in a food journal? Is it on track? Are you tracking every single calorie that passed your lips? (flavored water, vitamins, gum, single pieces of candy) Even if you aren't keeping track of calories, your body is!

- Are you eating too many calories?

- Are you eating too few calories?

- Are you taking in enough protein?

- Are the fats you're eating healthy (polyunsaturated and monounsaturated)?

- Are you eating too many simple carbohydrates (bread, pasta, potatoes, sugar, pasta, rice)

- Are you eating enough fruits and vegetables?

- Are you drinking enough water?

- Are you grazing?

- Are you eating the right quantity? Measuring and weighing foods?

- Are you eating on a schedule?

- Are you exercising hard enough? Long enough? Fast enough?

- When is the last time you changed your exercise routine? (The body becomes efficient and doesn't burn as many calories after you've done the same thing for four to six weeks.)

- Have you added weight training to your workouts? (Muscle burns more calories at rest.)

- Are you taking all your vitamins and supplements?

- Have you started taking any new medications that might promote weight gain?

- Have you taken your measurements (you might be losing inches even if the scale isn't moving)?

Maintenance is harder

Many of us have spent our entire lives, or at least our adult lives, trying to lose weight. How many years have we been obsessed with the next diet and begging the scale to move downward just another pound or two. Our world revolved around not being satisfied with ourselves.

Then along comes weight loss surgery and you're suddenly losing weight and fitting into clothes you never imagined wearing and approaching a goal weight. And you realize there's a real possibility that you'll keep the weight off that you never could keep off with any other diet you tried before. And then panic sets in. What do you do when you no longer need to lose weight? Many of us have never experienced this sensation before and you don't even know how to think or what to feel or what to do with your life when the scale no longer dictates your level of success.

What do you do when you no longer need to be on a weight loss plan and worry about losing weight?

The physical mechanics of maintaining a constant weight are fairly straightforward and any trained nutritionist can help you devise an eating plan to help you maintain the same weight on the scale. It's a simple matter of increasing your calorie intake to the same level as the number of calories you're expending and you stop losing weight. That's the easy part.

The hard part is wrapping your head around the idea that you no longer need to lose weight. The lifelong battle with the scale is over and you've finally won. But reversing 20 or 30 or 40 years of a diet-warrior mentality takes time and a new type of battle.

I wish I could give you a step-by-step plan for how to psychologically accept being in maintenance mode and moving on with the rest of your life. But there is no one set way to do that. Each person has a different battle to wage and your strategy won't be the same as my strategy or that of someone else's. Some important considerations might include:

Set many different types of goals early in your journey, not just weight or scale related goals. Find a new focus for your journey to health. Maybe it's time to try running a marathon or taking up a new hobby that you couldn't do when you were morbidly obese.

Enroll in a class or join an organization that will help you hone skills that contribute to your self-esteem such as Dale Carnegie classes or Toastmasters International club.

When you don't get to goal

My goal weight was "160-ish" - which meant that once my weight got into the 160's that I had achieved my goal. I always knew that 169 pounds was only my first goal weight and that when I achieved that weight I would set a new goal for a bit lower. In the back of my mind I always wanted to see 150 pounds but I wanted to set a conservative goal to begin with and play it safe. Little did I know that I'd never even see that initial conservative weight goal.

I stopped losing around 10 months post-op which was right in the midst of the period in time when I was training for a 10-mile race followed shortly by a half-marathon. The scale played games with me for a little while after that, but essentially the weight that I was at 10 months out, is the weight I'm at today. About 190 to 195 pounds.

I had my one year follow-up appointment about a month late, so at that point I'd been stalled for 3 months. My nutritionist and primary doctor didn't seem concerned and figured I'd start losing again any day. I got the standard speech about following the rules and sticking to the plan as prescribed (which I was).

I had my two year follow up appointment and the scale had then been stopped for 1 year and 3 months. Over the previous year I'd been wearing the GoWear Fit device (now called BodyMedia Fit) that measured my calorie output based on a number of scientific factors, so I knew how many calories I was burning. I had been experimenting with calorie intake (higher amounts, lower amounts) and nutrient content (more protein, less protein, more carbs, less carbs) and had switched up my exercises (walking, cycling, weight training). Nothing made the scale move either up or down.

My medical team was baffled. My primary doctor said to me: "You are doing everything right. I don't know what else to do for you." So he sent me to an endocrinologist who instantly put me on a prescription diet pill. After three months of pure hell that the pills caused I stopped taking them without any significant change in the scale (lost a few pounds, but they came back as soon as I stopped taking the pills).

About six months into my second year post-op I finally figured out that I needed to work on the mental side of things and find a way to accept the weight that I was and stop beating myself up about it. My body had a mind of its own and it was going to do whatever it wanted to do and I apparently had no control over it whatsoever. I'm still dealing with that emotional and mental battle but I feel like I'm in a much better place today than I was.

And now, here I am over five years after surgery and the scale still hasn't moved. It doesn't move up and it doesn't move down, no matter what I do or don't do. Sometimes I hate that bad behavior is not punished with added pounds and that good behavior is not rewarded with lost pounds. I've stopped trying to make the scale move and I'm just working on the psychological part of maintenance at this point. I've had to learn that following the rules isn't about seeing rewards on the scale or wearing smaller sized clothes. Following the rules of my surgery is about doing what's right for my body so I'm as healthy as possible on the inside.

Yes, it's frustrating when I can't make my body do what I want it to do. It's frustrating when I realize that I'm not in control of stuff (which is really hard when you're a control freak, like me). It's frustrating when doctors don't have the answers and when science can't tell us why the "calories in vs. calories out" theory doesn't work.

I don't know whether to be encouraged or discouraged that my situation is not unique or unusual. There are many WLS patients who never get to a goal weight they've set and have to adjust their mind set to accept a weight that is more than what they want it to be.

I've lost a total of 66% of my excess weight. We learned earlier that RNY patients will lose about 48% to 85% of their excess weight within the first two years post-op and maintain a loss of 53% to 77% at six years post-op. This means that I'm within the range of being a success according to the studies. But it has been difficult to accept my "measly" 66% next to some of my WLS friends who achieved 80% or 100%. Comparing my achievements to those of others is a dangerous game to start playing and it's something I work on not doing almost every day. Remember the wise saying: "Comparison is the thief of joy."

I don't intend for my story of never getting to my goal weight to discourage you. There are many more stories of success to look to where weight goals were triumphantly achieved, even after long plateaus. A dear friend of mine who had RNY a year before me, lost a significant amount of weight early in his post-op journey, but the scale stopped well before he reached his goal weight. After eight months at the same weight and being frustrated with the prolonged plateau, he made some major adjustments to his mental attitude, his eating plan, and exercise routine and suddenly the scale started moving again. He's an inspiration at our support group meetings and I admire his perseverance in finding a way to reach his weight goal.

Obviously, the scale can't be my full measure of success. Maybe I didn't hit my ultimate goal of 150 pounds but I've done an amazing job of becoming a healthier person and achieving all the other goals I've set for myself — including publishing this book. At some point we have to make the change from beating ourselves up over meaningless numbers on a plastic machine that lives in the bathroom next to the toilet. It's time to learn what to accept yourself as the amazing person you are.

No matter where you are in your own weight loss journey — achieving your ideal weight, not achieving it, or still struggling to get there — remember that measuring your success has a lot more to do with living a normal life and being happy with the person you are, than it does having a magic number appear on the scale.

The reality of regain

When we are newly post-op we have a very difficult time comprehending that anyone could eat enough food to ever gain the weight back after we lose it. Many times bariatric clinics don't adequately warn patients that regaining weight is a very real possibility and what steps to take to avoid that reality. Or maybe patients were warned by their surgical team but that information was blocked out while in the euphoric stage of rapid weight loss and the honeymoon phase.

Just so we don't misunderstand each other, here are the facts about weight loss and regain:[22]

Bariatric Procedure	Follow-up period		
	1-2 years	3-6 years	7-10 years
Gastric banding	29-87%	45-72%	14-60%
Sleeve Gastrectomy	33-58%	66%	-
Roux-en-Y gastric bypass	48-85%	53-77%	25-68%
Biliopancreatic diversion ± DS	65-83%	62-81%	60-80%

"But regain isn't possible since we can only eat small amounts of food at a time." This is a common misconception. Unfortunately it doesn't matter how small or big your stomach is after bariatric surgery, there are ways to pack in excess calories if you really want to. We are masters of dieting, remember? Or rather, we're masters of failing at dieting. And we also know how to bend the rules to suit our own justifications for bad behavior and we know how to delude ourselves into thinking we're not doing anything wrong.

Maybe you're not eating fast food triple decker burgers and mega size orders of french fries topped off with an extra-large Coke and dessert of a deep fried apple pie. No, a huge meal like that wouldn't fit into your small stomach all at one time without you noticing that you're overeating. But a couple handfuls of trail mix made of nuts, dried fruit and chocolate pieces would give you over 600 calories and you'd still have room for more in an hour or so. Or if you're eating that trail mix in tiny little servings — just a couple nuts at a time — you could polish off two or three cups of the mix over the course of the day simply be grazing on it little-by-little all day long.

There are a hundred — or a thousand — other ways to gain weight after WLS and they all can be traced back to our old habits of morbid obesity. We get lax in following the rules once we reach a year or two post-op. It's easy to let your guard down and revert back to what you've known all your life. Staying on track with the right eating plan, the right exercise routine and working on the psychological stuff is hard work and sometimes you get tired of all the effort it takes. But knowing from the beginning that regaining your lost weight — either all of it or some of it — is a reality you might need to face, you can start out being more diligent in your quest for better health.

If you find yourself regaining weight the only way to take it off again is to get back on the plan you're supposed to be following. There are myriad fad-diets being touted for bariatric patients — liquid fasts, pouch tests and all-protein style diets. But we know all too well that diets don't work. So you have to be very careful not to fall into the trap of trying the hottest new fad-diet when you start to see the scale creep up after WLS. Instead you need to focus your energies on following the rules you know are designed to work for post-op patients. Get back to basics.

Back to Basics

We hear it often "Back to Basics" but what does it really mean? Sometimes we get sidetracked with eating and exercise after WLS or during any weight loss plan and we need to get ourselves back on track with some basic rules and guidelines. These are the rules I think of when I hear the term "back to basics."

Support. Find a good in-person local support group. It can be a peer-based group like the one I lead in my hometown or it can be your surgeon's group meetings. Once you find a group to join, never miss a meeting. Make it a priority, put it on the calendar and don't let other things interfere with this important part of being successful. Statistics show that patients who attend in-person support group meetings have a higher rate of long term success in maintaining their weight loss[2]. I often tell my support group that the day you most feel like skipping your group meeting is the day when you probably need a meeting the most.

Follow your basic eating plan. You know the rules, you know how to use your tool, so do it.

Protein first and always. A good rule of thumb is "two bites of protein to one bite of something else." So that means even if an apple is a healthy snack, if you don't include a protein source with it, you're not following the rule of "protein first."

Practice moderation with carbohydrates. Focus on vegetables, fruit, dairy, legumes, and whole grains to get your carbohydrate needs. Avoid simple carbohydrates like white flour and sugar, pasta, rice, bread, and sweet treats. And remember to get enough fiber to keep the digestive tract working properly.

Get enough good fats in your diet. My goal is to have 25% of my calories coming from fat.

Choose dense meals, not sliders. Soft foods will slide straight through your pouch and leave you hungry sooner. Dense food, like a grilled chicken breast and vegetables, can stay in your pouch for up to two hours or until you start drinking water again.

Drink your fluids. Aim for a minimum of 64 ounces of water per day.

No drinking with meals or for 30-90 minutes after meals.

Track every morsel of food that passes your lips. You can't know how to adjust your intake unless you know where you are starting from. Figure out where your calories need to be and stick to it 90 percent of the time. Studies show that people who track calories lose more weight than those who don't.[23]

Plan your meals and eat on a schedule. I still follow the hour-by-hour schedule that I received in pre-surgical nutrition class which recommended three meals and two to three snacks, pre-planned, and eaten at specific times during the day and water intake between to curb hunger and grazing.

Vitamins. Be a religious fanatic about your vitamins and supplements.

Exercise your butt off. If you're not sweating like a pig, you're not working hard enough.

Plateaus. If the scale has stopped moving and you're in the midst of a plateau, make sure you review the list of questions to ask yourself in the section called Breaking a Stall.

Make sure you're healthy. If you haven't had labs drawn recently then get that done. Some vitamin deficiencies can actually cause weight gain so eliminating that as a culprit is important. Also take a close look at your medications list to determine if any of those be causing weight problems. Consult your doctors for help on these two considerations.

Lean on Others. When you're not strong enough to do it on your own, lean on others until you get your strength back. That's why the WLS support community is there. Eventually you will become strong enough and you can be the support person that someone else relies on down the road.

Get help if you need it. If you need to deal with the emotional struggles that go with food addiction and disordered eating and figuring out how to create a healthy relationship with food, then make an appointment with a therapist. A psychologist recommended by your surgeon's office is often the best resource. Find a doctor who is trained to work with weight loss surgery patients regarding eating disorders. You don't have to do it on your own.

You can do hard things! As my friend Shari said, you're worth the effort it takes to be healthy, happy and strong. You can do hard things.[23] Believe in yourself. And remember the words of Winston Churchill: "Never ever ever give in. Never give up."

Laughing in the Face of "Hard"

One of the sayings that WLS patients hate to hear is the accusation that we've taken the "easy way out." I personally believe that doing something the easy way isn't necessarily a bad thing. Why do it the hard way if the hard way doesn't work? Yes, bariatric surgery has allowed me to lose my excess weight in a fairly easy manner and the surgical tool that I have is something I'll always be able to rely on to help me maintain my weight loss. But just because losing the weight was fairly easy doesn't mean that this WLS journey has been easy. In fact, it's the hardest thing I've ever done in my life.

In the years since my bariatric surgery I have discovered just how strong of a person I really am. I have achieved goals and accomplished amazing feats that I never would have done before surgery. Going from morbid obesity to being a half-marathoner in less than a year. Going back to college to get my degree at 40 years old. Leading a support group and writing a book. Wow! Talk about laughing in the face of "hard" and coming out the victor.

Losing my excess weight through bariatric surgery might have been the easy way. Discovering my true self in the process was harder than I expected it to be but the rewards far outweigh the work it took to become a success in this Journey to a Healthier Me.

Resources
References • Links • Information

All the information, links, and resources listed in this section is also available on Pam's website. Please visit: **www.PamTremble.com/Journey**

Reference 1 • page 11
Diabetic patients had an overall 78.1% resolution of their clinical manifestations of diabetes, and diabetes was improved or resolved in 86.6% in the 621 bariatric patients studied. Diabetes resolution was greatest for patients undergoing biliopancreatic diversion/duodenal switch (95.1% resolved), followed by Roux-en-Y gastric bypass (80.3%), and then laparoscopic adjustable gastric banding (56.7%).

Buchwald H, Estok R, Fahrbach K, Banel D, Jensen MD, Pories WJ, Bantle JP, Sledge I: Weight and Type 2 Diabetes after Bariatric Surgery: Systematic Review and Meta-analysis. The American Journal of Medicine. Volume 122, Issue 3 , Pages 248-256.e5, March 2009.

Another source reports these rates for remission of type 2 diabetes mellitus after bariatric surgery:

Procedure	Remission Rate
Laparoscopic adjustable gastric banding	40–47
Roux-en-Y gastric bypass	83–92
Biliopancreatic diversion + DS	95–100

Mechanick, J. I., Kushner, R. F., Sugerman, H. J., Gonzalez-Campoy, J. M., Collazo-Clavell, M. L., Guven, S., ... & Dixon, J. (2008). American Association of Clinical Endocrinologists, The Obesity Society, and American Society for Metabolic & Bariatric Surgery Medical guidelines for clinical practice for the perioperative nutritional, metabolic, and nonsurgical support of the bariatric surgery patient. Endocrine Practice, 14, 1-83.

Reference 2 • page 14

Studies have shown that patients who attend support group meetings have a higher success rate for long term weight loss. Of the patients studied, those who attended support group meetings regularly had a statistically significant difference in percentage decrease of BMI compared to patients who didn't not attend meeting (42% vs. 32%).

Orth, W. S., Madan, A. K., Taddeucci, R. J., Coday, M., & Tichansky, D. S. (2008). Support group meeting attendance is associated with better weight loss. Obesity surgery, 18(4), 391-394.

Reference 3 • page 30

A randomized clinical trial evaluated the efficiency of intensive medical therapy alone versus bariatric surgery (Roux-en-Y gastric bypass or sleeve gastrectomy) in 150 obese patients with uncontrolled type 2 diabetes. Of the patients who underwent bariatric surgery, more than 60 percent had moderate-to-severe fatty liver disease on the basis of biopsy samples obtained during surgery.

Schauer, P. R., Kashyap, S. R., Wolski, K., Brethauer, S. A., Kirwan, J. P., Pothier, C. E., ... & Bhatt, D. L. (2012). Bariatric surgery versus intensive medical therapy in obese patients with diabetes. New England Journal of Medicine, 366(17), 1567-1576.

Reference 4 • page 31

For every 1% of your excess body weight you lose before surgery, studies show that you will have a 1.8% higher weight loss at 12-months post-op than those who did not lose weight pre-op. Plus, it's been shown that those who lose more than 5% of their excess weight will have a shorter operating time by 36 minutes. Conversely, weight gain before surgery comes with consequences. For every one unit on the BMI scale you increase your weight, you will lose 1.34% less weight than those who did not gain pre-op.

Alvarado, R., Alami, R. S., Hsu, G., Safadi, B. Y., Sanchez, B. R., Morton, J. M., & Curet, M. J. (2005). The impact of preoperative weight loss in patients undergoing laparoscopic Roux-en-Y gastric bypass. Obesity surgery, 15(9), 1282-1286.

Reference 5 • page 35

An average adult has 30 billion fat cells with a weight of 30 lbs. If excess weight is gained as an adult, fat cells increase in size about fourfold before dividing and increasing the absolute number of fat cells present.

Pool, Robert (2001). Fat: fighting the obesity epidemic. Oxford [Oxfordshire]: Oxford University Press. ISBN 0-19-511853-7.

Reference 6 • page 40

The average human stomach can hold up to two to four liters of food/fluid, that's about 52 ounces or 6½ cups! At rest your stomach is about the size of a man's fist but when filled with food and liquid it can expand to the size of a football.

Curtis, Helena & N. Sue Barnes. Invitation to Biology. 5th Edition. New York: Worth, 1994: 529.

Reference 7 • page 42

Studies have shown that the size of your pouch has very little to do with your overall success with weight loss. Your success has more to do with how well you follow your eating and exercise plan and how well you follow the rules of the pouch. Success depends on changing the way you live your life and the behavioral changes you make in the way you eat and think about food.

Bond, D., Leahey, T. M., Vithiananthan, S., & Ryder, B. (2009). Bariatric surgery for severe obesity: the role of patient behavior. Medicine and health, Rhode Island, 92(2), 58.

Reference 8 • page 41

Sites of nutrient absorption in the gastrointestinal tract diagram. Reprinted with permission.

Sareen S. Gropper, Jack L. Smith. Advanced Nutrition and Human Metabolism. Cengage Learning Nelson Education. Published February 14, 2008. ISBN-13: 978-0495116578. p 51.

Reference 9 • page 43

Although there are few human data, observations in animal models of short bowel syndrome have indicated that following massive enterectomy (surgical removal of a portion of the intestine), the bowel lengthens some and it increases in diameter. The number and size of intestinal villi increase, and therefore the absorptive surface area increases. This complete process is generally thought to occur over 1-2 years in humans, although there are isolated cases that have taken 5-7 years for adaptation.

Alan L. Buchman, MD, MSPH. Intestinal Adaptation Following Massive Enterectomy. Medscape General Medicine. 2004;6(2):12. Published online at: http://www.medscape.com/viewarticle/474629_2

Reference 10 • page 46

Dumping syndrome is a common side effect after Roux-en-Y Gastric Bypass surgery. About 85% of gastric bypass patients will experience dumping syndrome at some point after surgery. The symptoms can range from mild to severe.

The American Society for Metabolic and Bariatric Surgery (ASMBS). ASBS Public/ Professional Education Committee. Bariatric Surgery: Postoperative Concerns. Published: May 23, 2007. Revised February 7, 2008. Published online at: http://asmbs. org/2012/01/bariatric-surgery-postoperative-concerns/

Reference 11 • page 46

In persons with long segment Barrett esophagus treated with a truncal vagotomy, partial gastrectomy, plus Roux-en-Y gastrojejunostomy, 41% developed dumping within the first 6 months after surgery, but severe dumping is rare (5% of cases). Clinically significant dumping syndrome occurs in approximately 10% of patients after any type of gastric surgery.

Thomson, A. B., Padda, S., Ramirez, F., & Aguirre, T. (2008). Dumping syndrome. EMedicine Gastroenterology, 6, 1-6. Published online at: http://emedicine.medscape. com/article/173594-overview

Reference 12 • page 47

"Head Hunger is very real and even feels like real hunger, but if you are truly listening to your body (and not your head)... you will realize Head Hunger is that thing that makes you think you want to eat even when you know you're already full or when you know you have already eaten."

Tracy C., Barix Support Group Leader. Combating Head Hunger. Healthful Tips Newsletter. Copyright 2009. Forest Health Services.

Reference 13 • page 80

This ASMBS supplementation regimen is a part of the ASMBS Bariatric Nutrition report published in 2008. This information is intended for life-long daily supplementation for routine postoperative patients and is not intended to treat deficiencies. A patient's individual co-morbid conditions or changes in health status might require adjustments to this regimen.

American Society of Metabolic and Bariatric Surgeons (ASMBS). Bariatric Nutrition: Suggestions for Surgical Weight Loss Patients. Society of Obesity and Related Disease (SOARD) Publication . March 12, 2008. Published online at: http://s3.amazonaws.com/ publicASMBS/GuidelinesStatements/Guidelines/bgs_final.pdf

Reference 14 • page 83

Mean calcium absorption in the patients with achlorhydria was 0.452 (45%) for citrate and 0.042 (4%) for carbonate. Absorption of calcium from carbonate in patients with achlorhydria was significantly lower than in the normal subjects and was lower than absorption from citrate in either group; absorption from citrate in those with achlorhydria was significantly higher than in the normal subjects, as well as higher than absorption from carbonate in either group.

RR Recker. Calcium absorption and achlorhydria. New England Journal of Medicine. Volume 313:70-73, July 11, 1985.

Reference 15 • page 85

A cross-sectional survey was conducted on 144 patients of whom 80 had not undergone bariatric surgery, while 64 had bariatric surgery at a mean of 36 months previously. 25(OH)D levels were defined as being normal (>50 nmol/L), insufficient (2550 nmol/L) and deficient (<25 nmol/L). RESULTS: 80% of the patients presented low vitamin D levels.

Ybarra J, Sanchez-Hernandez J, Vich I, et al. Unchanged hypovitaminosis D and secondary hyperparathyroidism in morbid obesity alter bariatric surgery. Obes Surg 2005;15:330 –5.

Reference 16 • page 85

Ethnic minorities such as African-Americans have an increased risk of developing low vitamin D as a result of increased skin pigmentation conferring a natural sunscreen effect. A significant inverse correlation between 25OHD levels and BMI existed; 84.8% of all patients had vitamin D insufficiency and 75.8% had vitamin D deficiency. African-Americans were more likely to have hypovitaminosis D (95.5% vs. 60%) versus whites.

Dubin, R. L., Rasul, K., Allerton, T., Cefalu, W. T., Uwaifo, G. I., & Paige, J. T. Hypovitaminosis D in Patients Awaiting Weight-Loss Surgery in Southern Louisiana.

Reference 17 • page 85

D3 is approximately 87% more potent in raising and maintaining serum 25(OH)D concentrations and produces 2- to 3-fold greater storage of vitamin D than does equimolar D2. Given its greater potency and lower cost, D3 should be the preferred treatment option when correcting vitamin D deficiency.

Heaney, R. P., Recker, R. R., Grote, J., Horst, R. L., & Armas, L. A. (2011). Vitamin D3 is more potent than vitamin D2 in humans. Journal of Clinical Endocrinology & Metabolism, 96(3), E447-E452.

Reference 18 • page 85

The current government recommendation for Vitamin D intake for adults is 600iu per day.

Office of Dietary Supplements, National Institutes of Health. Dietary Supplement Fact Sheet: Vitamin D. January 24, 2011. Published online at: http://ods.od.nih.gov/factsheets/VitaminD-HealthProfessional/

Reference 19 • page 85

The Vitamin D Council was founded in 2003 by John J. Cannell, MD as a 501(c)(3) nonprofit organization, spreading reliable information on vitamin D, sun exposure and the vitamin D deficiency pandemic. The Vitamin D Council recommends the following amounts of supplemental vitamin D3 per day in the absence of proper sun exposure. These are only estimated amounts:

- Healthy children under the age of 1 years – 1,000 IU

- Healthy children over the age of 1 years – 1,000 IU per every 25 lbs of body weight

- Healthy adults and adolescents – at least 5,000 IU

- Pregnant and lactating mothers - at least 6,000 IU

The Vitamin D Council. Vitamin D Factsheet. As published online at: http://www.vitamindcouncil.org/about-vitamin-d/how-to-get-your-vitamin-d/vitamin-d-supplementation/

Reference 20 • page 86

Emerging science is showing that Vitamin D lab results above 50nmol/L or above 20 ng/mL are helping patients realize many amazing health benefits such as reduced risk of certain cancers, inflammation leading to chronic diseases and a reduced risk of developing neuromuscular diseases such as muscular dystrophy.

Office of Dietary Supplements, National Institutes of Health. Dietary Supplement Fact Sheet: Vitamin D. January 24, 2011. Published online at: http://ods.od.nih.gov/factsheets/VitaminD-HealthProfessional/

Reference 21 • page 92

The chart entitled Common Vitamin Deficiencies is a compilation of information I've gathered over the past five or six years from various sources on the internet, in medical journals, nutrition textbooks, and publications provided by various bariatric surgical practices. I was not the original creator the framework and I'm unable to identify the original source because it is published, in one form or another, on many different websites by many different people or organizations. The original chart has changed since I got my hands on it and added information as I researched various nutrient topics. My version of the chart has been online for several years, so it's difficult to determine if all the sources listed below contain original information or if the information was gleaned from mine.

However, please know that I'm publishing this chart as an informational tool and do not wish to infringe on anyone's copyrighted information. To the best of my knowledge, the information compiled in this chart either comes from these online sources or is additionally referenced on these websites:

World's Healthiest Foods: www.whfoods.com

Lab Results Online: www.labtestsonline.org

Changing Shape: www.changingshape.com/resources/references/vmchart.php

National Review of Medicine: www.nationalreviewofmedicine.com/issue/what_tell_patients/2007/4_tell_patients_3.html

1st Holistic Nutrition: www.1stholistic.com/nutrition/hol_nutr-def-symptoms.htm

Reference 22 • page 135

The purpose of bariatric surgery is to induce substantial, clinically important weight loss that is sufficient to reduce obesity related medical complications to acceptable levels.

Bariatric Procedure	Follow-up period		
	1-2 years	3-6 years	7-10 years
Gastric banding	29-87%	45-72%	14-60%
Sleeve Gastrectomy	33-58%	66%	-
Roux-en-Y gastric bypass	48-85%	53-77%	25-68%
Biliopancreatic diversion ± DS	65-83%	62-81%	60-80%

Mechanick, J. I., Kushner, R. F., Sugerman, H. J., Gonzalez-Campoy, J. M., Collazo-Clavell, M. L., Guven, S., ... & Dixon, J. (2008). American Association of Clinical Endocrinologists, The Obesity Society, and American Society for Metabolic & Bariatric Surgery Medical guidelines for clinical practice for the perioperative nutritional, metabolic, and nonsurgical support of the bariatric surgery patient. Endocrine Practice, 14, 1-83.

Reference 23 • page 137

Among adults who reported losing weight or trying to lose weight, 31.0% had been successful at both losing weight and maintenance after weight loss. Assessment of reported weight loss strategies, found that exercising ≥30 minutes/day and adding physical activity to daily life were significantly higher among successful versus unsuccessful weight losers. Significantly more successful versus unsuccessful weight losers reported that on most days of the week they planned meals (35.9% vs. 24.9%), tracked calories (17.7% vs. 8.8%), tracked fat (16.4% vs. 6.6%), and measured food on plate (15.9% vs. 6.7%). Successful losers were also more likely to weigh themselves daily (20.3% vs. 11.0%).

Kruger, J., Blanck, H. M., & Gillespie, C. (2006). Dietary and physical activity behaviors among adults successful at weight loss maintenance. International Journal of Behavioral Nutrition and Physical Activity, 3(1), 17.

Reference 24 • page 138

The essay "I can do hard things!" was written by Shari (aka Jupiter6 on ObesityHelp.com) as a forum thread. It quickly went viral within the WLS community and became the mantra for many of us as we persevered in the face of hard things. You can read the entire essay at: www.PamTremble.com/journey

Resources • Links • Information

Stories of Fellow WLS'ers

There are many bariatric patients online who are chronicling their journey to health. I have found inspiration through these people and I hope you do too. Please visit their websites to read real life stories of others in our weight loss surgery community.

Nikki | Bariatric Foodie
www.bariatricfoodie.com

Michelle | The World According to Eggface
www.theworldaccordingtoeggface.com

Beth | Melting Mama & Bariatric Bad Girls
www.MeltingMama.net

Rob | Former Fat Dudes
www.FormerFatDudes.com

Andrea | WLS Vitagarten
www.wlsvitagarten.com

Online Support Communities

Obesity Help | www.ObesityHelp.com

WLS Boards | www.wlsboards.com

Thinner Times | www.ThinnerTimesForum.com

Connection WLS | www.ConnectionWLS.com

WLS Journey | www.WLSJourney.org

iVillage | www.forums.ivillage.com (search "weight loss surgery support")

Finding Protein Powder Samples

Vitalady | www.vitalady.com

Netrition | www.netrition.com

Nashua Nutrition | www.nashuanutrition.com

Chike | www.chikenutrition.com

Click | www.drinkclick.com

Unjury | www.unjury.com

The Minnesota Starvation Study

The symptoms I experienced in the early days of my pre-op diet - and in the months after my surgery - are typical of people who severely restrict calorie intake. Obsessive thoughts of food and obsessive preoccupation with any topic related to food were common in the study participants during WWII.

Read the full accounting of the study at: jn.nutrition.org/cgi/content/full/135/6/1347

38874438R00088

Made in the USA
Middletown, DE
29 December 2016